A Conceptual Framework for SMART Applications in Higher Education:

Emerging Research and Opportunities

James Orion Connelly
University of Phoenix, USA

Paula Miller
University of Phoenix, USA

A volume in the Advances in Higher Education and Professional Development (AHEPD) Book Series

IGI Global
DISSEMINATOR OF KNOWLEDGE

Published in the United States of America by
IGI Global
Information Science Reference (an imprint of IGI Global)
701 E. Chocolate Avenue
Hershey PA, USA 17033
Tel: 717-533-8845
Fax: 717-533-8661
E-mail: cust@igi-global.com
Web site: http://www.igi-global.com

Library of Congress Cataloging-in-Publication Data

Names: Miller, Paula, 1954- author. | Connelly, James Orion, 1943- author.
Title: A conceptual framework for SMART applications in higher education : emerging research and opportunities / by Paula Miller and James Orion Connelly.
Description: Hershey, PA : Information Science Reference, 2020. | Includes bibliographical references and index. | Summary: "This book explores how teaching and learning can be made more efficient and effective through the use of SMART applications in higher education"-- Provided by publisher.
Identifiers: LCCN 2019030359 (print) | LCCN 2019030360 (ebook) | ISBN 9781799815426 (hardcover) | ISBN 9781799815433 (paperback) | ISBN 9781799815440 (ebook)
Subjects: LCSH: Cognitive neuroscience. | Neuroplasticity. | Education, Higher--Effect of technological innovations on. | Information retrieval--Technological innovations.
Classification: LCC QP360.5 .M537 2020 (print) | LCC QP360.5 (ebook) | DDC 612.8/233--dc23
LC record available at https://lccn.loc.gov/2019030359
LC ebook record available at https://lccn.loc.gov/2019030360

This book is published in the IGI Global book series Advances in Higher Education and Professional Development (AHEPD) (ISSN: 2327-6983; eISSN: 2327-6991)

British Cataloguing in Publication Data
A Cataloguing in Publication record for this book is available from the British Library.

For electronic access to this publication, please contact: eresources@igi-global.com.

Advances in Higher Education and Professional Development (AHEPD) Book Series

ISSN:2327-6983
EISSN:2327-6991

Editor-in-Chief: Jared Keengwe, University of North Dakota, USA

MISSION

As world economies continue to shift and change in response to global financial situations, job markets have begun to demand a more highly-skilled workforce. In many industries a college degree is the minimum requirement and further educational development is expected to advance. With these current trends in mind, the **Advances in Higher Education & Professional Development (AHEPD) Book Series** provides an outlet for researchers and academics to publish their research in these areas and to distribute these works to practitioners and other researchers.

AHEPD encompasses all research dealing with higher education pedagogy, development, and curriculum design, as well as all areas of professional development, regardless of focus.

COVERAGE

- Adult Education
- Assessment in Higher Education
- Career Training
- Coaching and Mentoring
- Continuing Professional Development
- Governance in Higher Education
- Higher Education Policy
- Pedagogy of Teaching Higher Education
- Vocational Education

IGI Global is currently accepting manuscripts for publication within this series. To submit a proposal for a volume in this series, please contact our Acquisition Editors at Acquisitions@igi-global.com or visit: http://www.igi-global.com/publish/.

The Advances in Higher Education and Professional Development (AHEPD) Book Series (ISSN 2327-6983) is published by IGI Global, 701 E. Chocolate Avenue, Hershey, PA 17033-1240, USA, www.igi-global.com. This series is composed of titles available for purchase individually; each title is edited to be contextually exclusive from any other title within the series. For pricing and ordering information please visit http://www.igi-global.com/book-series/advances-higher-education-professional-development/73681. Postmaster: Send all address changes to above address.

Titles in this Series

For a list of additional titles in this series, please visit:
https://www.igi-global.com/book-series/advances-higher-education-professional-development/73681

Culturally Responsive Teaching and Learning in Higher Education
Lucretia Octavia Tripp (Auburn University, USA) and Rhonda M. Collier (Tuskegee University, USA)
Information Science Reference • copyright 2020 • 350pp • H/C (ISBN: 9781522599890) • US $195.00 (our price)

Examining the Role of Entrepreneurial Universities in Regional Development
Ana Dias Daniel (University of Aveiro, Portugal) Aurora A.C. Teixeira (Universidade do Porto, Portugal) and Miguel Torres Preto (Universidade de Lisboa, Portugal)
Business Science Reference • copyright 2020 • 360pp • H/C (ISBN: 9781799801740) • US $215.00 (our price)

IT Issues in Higher Education Emerging Research and Opportunities
Lazarus Ndiku Makewa (Rwenzori International University, Kenya) and Baraka Manjale Ngussa (University of Arusha, Tanzania)
Information Science Reference • copyright 2020 • 169pp • H/C (ISBN: 9781799810292) • US $165.00 (our price)

Effects of Engagement and Resources on Learning Outcomes in Vocational Colleges Emerging Research and Opportunities
Joseph Muthiani Malechwanzi (Pwani University, Kenya)
Information Science Reference • copyright 2020 • 188pp • H/C (ISBN: 9781522592501) • US $145.00 (our price)

Emerging Perspectives on Community Schools and the Engaged University
Robert F. Kronick (University of Tennessee, USA)
Information Science Reference • copyright 2020 • 307pp • H/C (ISBN: 9781799802808) • US $195.00 (our price)

For an entire list of titles in this series, please visit:
https://www.igi-global.com/book-series/advances-higher-education-professional-development/73681

IGI Global
DISSEMINATOR OF KNOWLEDGE

701 East Chocolate Avenue, Hershey, PA 17033, USA
Tel: 717-533-8845 x100 • Fax: 717-533-8661
E-Mail: cust@igi-global.com • www.igi-global.com

Table of Contents

Preface

We live in an exciting time of momentous change and in a literal explosion of information. The issue becomes one of meeting the challenge of rapidly accumulating information and turning that information into knowledge that benefits humanity. This need stimulated a search for a conceptual framework that could guide the use of instructional technology in education. The book is not intended to be a scientific treatise but is meant to be put to practical use in higher education. The book offers a conceptual framework to guide the application of instructional technology to keep pace with the information explosion by making instruction more effective and more efficient.

THE CHALLENGES

The primary challenge is to try to keep pace with the information explosion. The secondary challenge is to turn this information into useful knowledge. This raises the question: How can we do this? Neuroscience is one approach that is based on how the brain operates. We are discovering increasingly more about how this happens. Over the centuries and through observation and trial and error we already knew a good bit about how we teach and learn, but now we can verify this with scientific facts and discover previously unknown aspects of brain physiology. These observations of brain functioning have produced many learning theories, all of which have varying degrees of validity. These theories, in turn, gave birth to theories and models of instructional design, which also have varying degrees of validity.

Technology gives humanity the means through which they can see what is hidden from the eye and from the ear and gives us the opportunity to see and hear that which is far away or too small. This technology makes heavy use of computers and the way they work. Artificial intelligence is one way to sift through the exponential growth of data and to help generate knowledge from this ever-accumulating information.

SEARCHING FOR A SOLUTION

These challenges must be met. The problem is that the capacity of the mind is relatively static while the growth of information is exponential. This creates a profound imbalance, but one that can be partially addressed by learning more about how humans learn and manipulating those variables to produce more learning. Among these potential solutions is the growing sophistication of artificial intelligence. Appropriate algorithms of increasing sophistication will no doubt be devised to help bring order out of this confusing mass of information through artificial intelligence.

The overriding concern about instructional technology is that it must be applied in the context of sound pedagogic principles. While there are quite a few learning theories and instructional design models, one stands out above the rest: Gagné's nine instructional events, which is covered in chapter five, Table 12, and figures six, eight, and nine. This provides a sound pedagogy that serves many learning theories and instructional design models.

ORGANIZATION OF THE BOOK

This book is organized into four sections: "The Foundation," "The Elements," "The Future," and "Examples." "The Foundation" consists of basic topics: the information explosion; how we know the external world; and how memories are formed, stored, and retrieved. Section 2, "The Elements," consists of three topics: theories of learning, theories and models of instructional design;, and learner characteristics. Section 3, "The Future," consists of three topics: evolving instructional technology, tying it together, and the future of education. Section 4 consists of one single topic: the application of what we have learned that consists of four examples of application to academic courses.

Please note that each section and each chapter begin with a graphic organizer that shows the place of the section and the place of the chapter within the section in the overall structure of the book. This literary device provides continuity and structure to the volume.

Introduction

The information explosion and the glut of data it is producing has reached a bottleneck: more information than we can process. To compound the problem, the doubling of information is occurring at ever shorter intervals. It is estimated that the doubling will begin to take place every 12 hours. Realizing that it took more than 1,000 years for information double at the beginning of human history, this is indeed remarkable. Who knows what possibilities for a better world and a better life may slip by unnoticed, buried in the flood of information swept away unseen? Of course, evil events, as well, can slip away before they are enacted. Nevertheless, we miss and shall miss more wonderful opportunities that could arise from information that was not processed. How can we identify and make use of such information that holds considerable promise for humanity? Perhaps, it cannot be done, but we can become more efficient and effective at finding, identifying, and using helpful information. One approach is through education; however, a new paradigm must be found to guide teaching and learning before education can be of more value to us. This is the purpose of this book. The proposed conceptual framework could provide a launching point for research into how we can learn to cope with the information explosion and the changes to be shaped by it.

James O. Connelly
University of Phoenix, USA

Section 1
The Foundation

Section 1 lays the foundation for the purpose of this book. It is to find a way to make learning more effective and more efficient. This section deals with the information explosion, which lays the foundation for the purpose of the book. Chapter 2 concerns how we know the world external to us. This knowledge is arrived at via the five senses: sight, sound, taste, touch, and smell. Further, the senses are quite limited in what they are capable of perceiving, Consequently, we have invented devices that let us capture what is beyond our ability to perceive with our natural senses. These devices include radio, telephone, satellite communication, television, and the microscope. As Shakespeare so aptly observed as expressed through his character, Hamlet, "There are more things in heaven and earth, Horation, than are dreampt of in your philosophy." Further are explored what we are learning about how the brain works, memory, the influence of emotions, neuroplasticity, neurogenesis, cognitive load, schemata, SMART characteristics, student, administrative, and motivational characteristics. Examples are provided at the end of each chapter.

Figure 1.

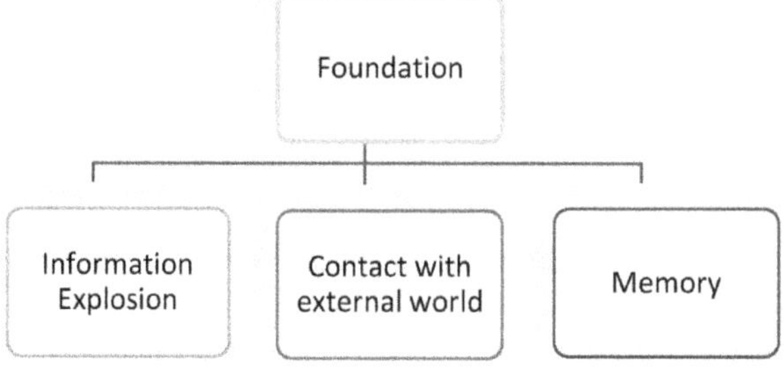

Chapter 1
The Information Explosion

ABSTRACT

This chapter lays the foundation for the conceptual framework by providing a background of the information explosion. The growth of information is examined from the year 1 AD to 2018 AD. The information explosion produced four major revolutions with intermediate contributions. The four information revolutions were identified by Peter Drucker as the invention of writing, the book, the printing press, and the computer age. This growth is delineated by the years in which information doubled. He compared the advent of the printing press (information revolution three) to the coming of age of the computer and the internet (the fourth of the four information revolutions). Each information revolution generated the need for allied industries. The massive growth of information may be coped with by becoming more effective and efficient learners and teachers.

THE KNOWLEDGE EXPLOSION

The accumulation of information and the knowledge derived from it has been growing so rapidly that it resembles an explosion. Information is growing exponentially. As information is generated and accumulated at an ever-accelerating rate, it becomes increasingly difficult to turn this vast quantity of information into knowledge. It reminds one of the Jerry Reed song *East Bound and Down* in which the lyrics state "We've got a long way to go and a short time to get there." We have much to learn and with no appreciable increase in brainpower or information processing capacity. The very nature

DOI: 10.4018/978-1-7998-1542-6.ch001

Figure 1.

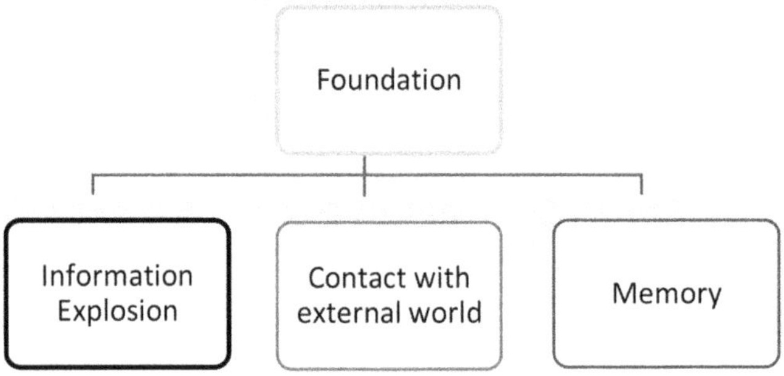

of the information explosion demands that one finds a way to make learning more effective and efficient in the hope of making the most of that information and turn it into knowledge. Artificial intelligence can help find and make some degree of sense of it.

KNOWLEDGE DOUBLING

The knowledge doubling curve, attributed to R. Buckminster Fuller in 1982 Lundell (2014) estimated that accumulated and transmitted human knowledge doubled in the year one AD. Another doubling took place about 1,500 years later. Then, another doubling occurred in about 250 years, in 1750. Yet another doubling happened in 1900, 150 years later. Current guesses at the beginning of the 21st century estimate the doubling to take place in one or two years. By 2017 the doubling was estimated to occur in approximately 12 hours (see Figure 2). Whether one agrees with these estimates is less important than the realization that there is an exponential growth rate in the accumulated information of humanity.

The computer and the Internet are not the first information revolution. Peter Drucker (1998) asserts that there were four information revolutions: the invention of writing, the book, the printing press, and the computer coupled with the Internet. With respect to the printing revolution, Drucker (1998) notes that

The most important lesson of the earlier information revolution may, however, be found in the fates and fortunes of its technologists. The printing revolution immediately created a new and unprecedented class of information

technologists, just as the most recent information revolution has created any number of information businesses, MIS and IT specialists, software designers, and chief information officers. The IT people of the printing revolution were the early printers. Nonexistent—and indeed not even imaginable—in 1455, they flourished throughout Europe 25 years later and had become great stars. Unlike earlier craftsmen, they were great gentlemen. These virtuosi of the printing press were known and revered all over Europe, just as the names of the leading computer and software firms are recognized and admired worldwide today. Printers were courted by kings, princes, the pope, and rich merchant cities and were showered with money and honors. ...Is there a lesson in this for today's information technologists, the CIOs in organizations, the software designers and developers, the devotees of Moore's Law? (pp. 8-9).

With the recognition that the aforementioned information revolutions had significant repercussions, it must be noted that other events contributed to the information explosion. The following table (Table 1) represents the view of the authors of *Timelines of History: The ultimate visual guide to the events that shaped the world. Second edition*, which provides one view of the knowledge explosion of which the invention of writing, the book, and printing are only three instances, but nevertheless important ones (The Smithsonian, 2018).

From the beginning of the Classical Age to the end of that age, there are 1,299 years (700BC to 1499AD). Within these centuries there are 913 significant events. Though the growth of knowledge is not overtly dealt with, one can extrapolate the growth of human knowledge from the growth of other factors. For example, the growth of the human population over a period of 4,000 years shows a dramatic upturn that closely follows a similar pattern as that shown in Figure 2. The use of fossil fuels presents a parallel pattern. Using population growth and the growth of fossil fuels as only two of several measures, it becomes evident that an increase in human knowledge is responsible for this growth. There could be as many views of the information explosion as there are individuals and institutions who think about such matters. At any rate, the foregoing arguments should illustrate the rapid growth of knowledge. Figure 2 represents this phenomenon:

To interpret the graph, let us assume that two units of information exist in the year one AD. If knowledge begins to double in about 1500, the initial two units would double to four units. Between 250 and 300 years later (1750 to 1800), knowledge doubles once again. At which time the four units would become eight units. Between 1800 and 1900 another doubling would occur and bring the units to 16. Things changed in 1900 because of an uptick in

Table 1. Table of contents copied from timelines of history to illustrate the growth of knowledge

Title	When	Features
Human Origins	8 MYA* to 3000 BC	Colonizing the Planet
		Prehistoric Peoples
Early Civilizations	3000BC to 300BC	The Story of Writing
		Ancient Empires
		Ancient Egypt
The Classical Age	700BC to 599BC	Ancient Greece
		The Story of Metal Working
		The Story of Money
		The Rise of the Roman Empire
		Ancient Rome
		Classical Trade
Trade and Invention	600 to 1499	The Vikings
		The Islamic World
		The Aztecs, Incas, and Maya
		The Story of Printing
Reformation & Exploration	1450 to 1749	Voyages of Exploration
		The Story of Astronomy
		Edo Period
		Mughal Empire
		The Renaissance
		The Story of Arms and Armor
		Rise and Fall of the Ottoman Empire
		The Story of Navigation
		The Story of Agriculture
The Age of Revolution	1750 to 1913	European Nation States
		The Story of Steam Power
		The Story of Medicine
		American Indians
		The Story of Electricity
		The American Civil War
		The Story of the Car

continued on following page

Table 1. Continued

Title	When	Features
Technology & Superpowers	1914 to 2018	The Great War
		Soviet Propaganda
		World War I
		The Story of Flight
		The Story of Communication
		War in Europe
		War in the Pacific
		World War II
		The Space Race
		End of Empire
		The Story of Genetics
		The collapse of the USSR
		The European Union
		Global Economy

* MYA = million years ago
The Smithsonian, (2018)

Figure 2. The rate at which information has doubled from 1AD to 2017

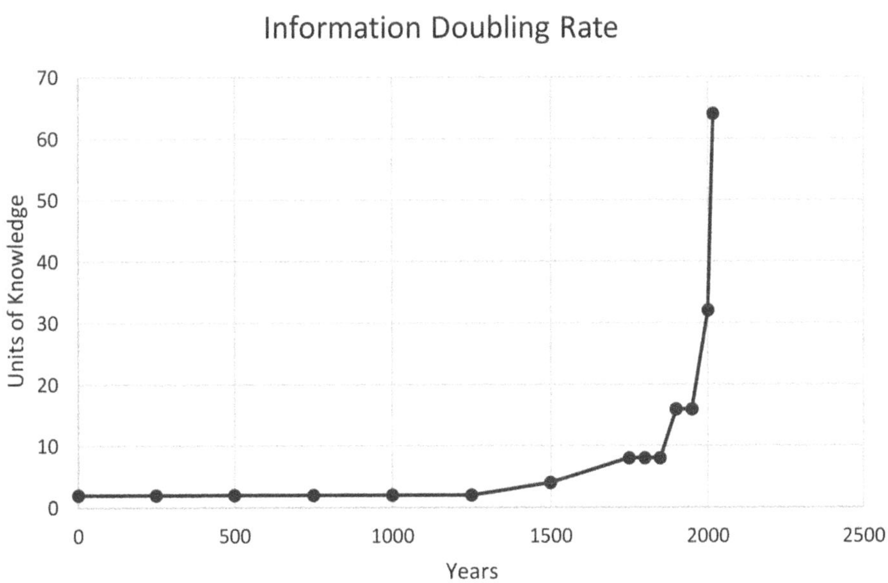

population growth, inventions, technology, and similar areas that snowballed until and through the beginning of the 21st century and continues apace. At the end of World War II, another doubling took place. Within a short space of time, the doubling began to occur at increasingly shorter intervals, until it was estimated that such doublings occurred in 12 months. Looking toward the future, it is estimated that the growth of human knowledge could double every two hours.

GROWTH OF ALLIED INDUSTRIES

With the advent of new technology or invention, a multitude of supporting occupations and systems emerged. For example, consider the printing press. As this new technology gained hold in Europe in the middle 1400s, William Caxton (Encyclopaedia Britannica, n.d.), then living in London, England, began to print books in the vernacular (English). This new technology created many unexperienced issues for printers. For example, William Caxton had to invent English spelling. Before then, Latin was the preferred international language of religion, education, science, the arts, and other fields. At that time, many dialects were spoken across England, as was the case in the languages of other countries. Caxton did business in London; therefore, that was the dialect that he chose for his books. This creating of spelling in English, in part, explains some of our strange spellings of words that once mirrored their pronunciation as enough, night, thought, and so forth. Apparently, a written language is perhaps less likely to change rapidly owing to the conventions of spelling. Today, owing to the widespread coverage of the mass media, particularly television, radio, and the spoken word on the Internet, a uniformity of pronunciation is ensured. Therefore, regional dialects seem to be declining as uniform speech slowly replaces them.

A similar example is the Chickasaw and Choctaw languages of the Native American tribes in Mississippi and Oklahoma. The Chickasaw tribe among others was removed to Oklahoma in the early 1830s. A significant number of that tribe escaped the removal and remained in Mississippi. The Chickasaws had no written language; therefore, there were no linguistic standards that governed written language, which seems to retard the rate of linguistic change. So, between the time of the removal in the mid-1830s and 1930 for example, the language changed. Now, the two branches of the Chickasaws can still understand one another, but there are differences that occurred because of their physical separation.

Returning to our example of William Caxton and the printing press we must consider how this tremendous technological advance influenced the growth of new occupations and the demise of others. The new printing industry required printing presses, the manufacture of paper and ink, education to help new learners to read, the distribution of books and other printed material. This advance led to the downfall of the occupations of those talented monks who laboriously hand-copied and illuminated various books. Further, the rapid production of books reduced vastly the cost of acquiring books and building personal libraries.

The example of the printing press points out how the technology improved to reach the massive standards of today. Once the concept of printing using moveable type was grasped, other individuals saw ways to improve on the process. Each generation contributed to printing improvement. The same phenomena can apply to the steam engine. Just imagine the first locomotives and compare them to the ones we have today. Likewise, the harnessing of electricity tells a similar story. The same circumstances occur within such diverse fields as transportation, agriculture, manufacturing, and the list could continue in a similar manner.

Over the millennia, humankind has been increasing in number. This is likely due to our species ability to generate information, turn it into knowledge, and apply that knowledge to our benefit. This creation of knowledge began slowly and continued slowly until the beginning of the 1900s. Since then, information has grown exponentially from a doubling once a century to anticipated doubling every 12 hours. This does have all the signs, indications, and features of an ever-increasing explosion of information and subsequent knowledge. The question arises: How can we cope with it? We must make learning more efficient and effective.

COPING WITH THE EXPLOSION OF INFORMATION

The problem becomes one of how to cope with this vast explosion of information. If we look at the situation as one that is characterized by a relatively static capacity of the brain to process, analyze, connect, and store new information, one must consider ways to make this activity more efficient and effective. Three options come to mind: 1) use of instructional technology, 2) more effective ways of designing instruction, and 3) presenting information in a way that recognizes how the brain works. Instructional technology can make use of all those advances in telecommunication technology and in computing technology. Presenting snippets of instruction via mobile digital devices make learning anytime, anywhere feasible. Cloud computing and storage make it possible to use software that does not reside on one's personal device. The personal device can then be used to navigate and interact with highly sophisticated programs while eliminating the need for massive memory capacity on personal computing and telecommunication devices.

Through improved instructional design methods, one could reduce the time it takes to learn and help make what is learned easier to comprehend, store in, and retrieve from long term memory. Current technology allied with good instructional design can provide feedback that is necessary for the process of learning. This feedback can be used formatively and summatively. Formatively, immediate feedback can be provided by branching to alternate screens that depend upon the learner's initial responses to prompts. These can be in the form of quizzes that both test and instruct. The instructive power lies in the immediate response to elements presented in the instructional program that keeps the learner on the path to knowledge. Summatively, instructional technology can identify areas in which the student is weak and requires review. Also, data can be recorded that helps the designers improve upon their designs.

One could expect that presenting information in a way that is compatible with what is being learned and how the brain operates could make learning more effective and more efficient. For example, the brain likes to reflect upon that with which it has been presented; therefore, by providing time for learners to journal or otherwise engage in active reflection could be expected to strengthen their learning of a lesson. It takes time for likeminded neurons to seek and find each other and form new connections or matrices; therefore, provide time for review and practice to strengthen those new ties. The attention span of the brain is relatively short; therefore, allow breaks and novel stimuli to refocus interest. The brain requires nourishment and oxygen to perform at its best; therefore, tell learners that they must eat healthy food and exercise to keep their brains in top form.

A NEW CONCEPTUAL FRAMEWORK

A new conceptual framework that recognizes all these elements is needed to cope with the information explosion. Figure 3 presents such a framework.

This conceptual framework begins before one confronts the diagram; it begins with what is to be taught and to whom it is to be taught. Then

Figure 3. A conceptual framework for coping with the information explosion

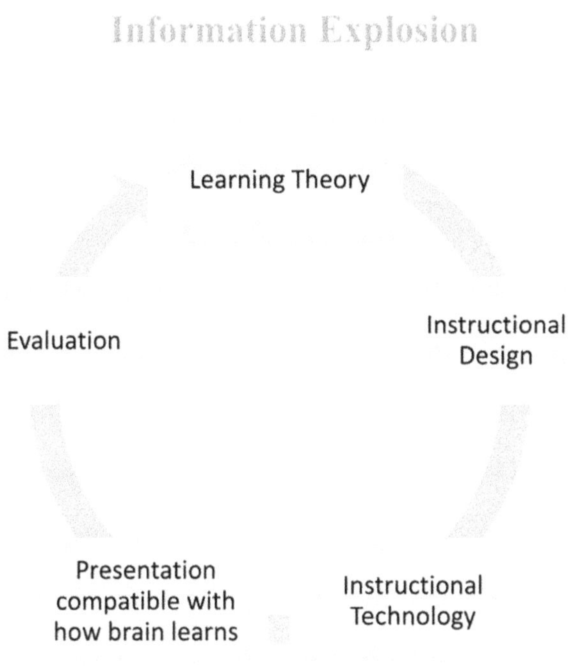

one begins at the top by selecting a learning theory. This selection will be determined by the nature of the content and the nature of the learners. A theory can be selected from the four major theories (i.e. behaviorist, cognitivist, constructivist, connectivist), or any of the other learning theories of which there are approximately 100 (David, 2017). The learning theory along with the content, the target audience, and the proposed delivery method will determine which instructional design model to use for guiding the presentation of the content. Instructional technology will help the designer to apply the design. This design must be one that exploits what is known about how the brain learns and operates. The final step is to evaluate the program, which is based on testing it on learners who match the characteristics of the target audience. After this, one uses formative and summative evaluation to make appropriate revisions to the instructional material and methods as they are needed. See more about this in chapters 4 and 5.

Now, it is time to select an instructional design model and a learning theory to govern the teaching and learning. Gagne's nine instructional events (Gagné, 1985) provide a solid foundation for designing a lesson. The learning theory to be used is dictated by the nature of the subject matter and the nature of the students. A taxonomy of educational objectives such as those created by Benjamin Bloom (cognitive), Krathwohl (affective), and Simpson (psychomotor) can provide guidance. For example, the level of learning can be established by the hierarchy of objectives presented in all three domains as expressed by the instructional objectives that are based on them.

After all this preparation, it is time to embark on creating the instructional content. This will be determined by the instructional objectives. The iterative nature of this model is such that if we modify, add, or remove an objective, the instructional content must also be modified to reflect the changes in the objectives. It is a complex process with considerable intertwining and subsequent modifications. Once all is done, it is time to beta test it to see how well it works before releasing the material for widespread use.

EXAMPLES

Examine the benefits that the information explosion has brought to four academic disciplines in higher education. History, science, literature, and archaeology were chosen because they are representative of areas of the curriculum found in most liberal arts universities.

History

The information explosion has produced both technology and content that furthers the exploration and learning of history. One may attempt to teach history from the human perspective of daily life. For this example, create a unit to present the Southern Perspective of the War Between the States. The technology needed for this would be that which permits access to the Internet to obtain and use digital recordings, photographs, video, and short instructional sequences with appropriate feedback and guidance ability.

On the Internet, one can access various links on the world wide web. This access could cross different technological platforms so that the material could be played back on personal computers, laptops, and an array of portable digital devices. To make this more efficient and effective, this access should be via learning management systems (LMSs) that are user-friendly. To save space on receptive digital devices, the material would be housed in the cloud.

Digital recordings are an effective way to record, store, and replay digital data. For example, a study of popular music of the period could be received, heard, and analyzed. During this period, death was a constant in the life of everyone: death from disease, in childbirth, accidents, and the War Between the States, which claimed about 750,000 lives of young men on both sides of the struggle ("Civil War Casualties", n.d.). The songs could be input into speech recognition software and transcribed to permit an analysis by such programs as Nvivo. The accountability movement has generated such programs for closed captioning of video material. This software could be used in the song analysis project.

Photographs of that period exist in great numbers, although the exposure times required for a print were excessively long by today's standards. These hauntingly beautiful photographic portraits of sweethearts, wives, husbands, children, soldiers give a face to the war and its enduring tragedy. Matthew Brady and others took pictures of battlefields and the casualties of war. The various leaders of both sides have left photographic images of themselves. Video sequences with synchronized audio can illustrate events from those years. Teachers can create instructional sequences using various kinds of authoring programs, even PowerPoint can serve as a shell or box in which to embed audio, video, still images, and basic animations.

Teaching applications can include WebQuests in which students locate the music of the period, photographs and hand-drawn illustrations from contemporaneous magazines, such as *Harper's Weekly*. Firsthand accounts by persons on both sides of the conflict are in various places on the Internet. These would make excellent collaborative projects for teams of students assigned to examine various aspects of the assignment within the context of constructivist learning theory.

Science

Thanks to the growth of technology and computers, one can see things that are incapable of being seen in the past; things that exceed the human ability to perceive without technological intervention. Examples are many: microscopes to see the very small, telescopes to see the very distant, audio manipulation that permits us to hear things below and above the threshold of our senses, and video manipulation to permit us to see colors that fall below and exist above what the eye can naturally perceive. One can statistically analyze data to help students and academics to arrive at conclusions that were not possible in years past.

The nature of action potentials via this new and developing technology can be explored. Living bodies are powered by electrical impulses that are generated in neurons, transmitted along axons and across synaptic spaces to other neurons or muscles. These action potentials are generated by the exchange of sodium and potassium ions through cell membranes. Once the threshold has been reached (typically between a negative 50 and negative 55 millivolts), the neuron fires an electrical impulse (Despopoulos, A., & Silbernagle, S., 1983. P. 30). This phenomenon, owing to the threshold value, creates an all or nothing response; zeros and ones, which make it a digital signal.

Through special microscopes and electronic devices, scientists can now see the firing of these impulses. To see an example, use this search term *video of calcium signaling* and prepare to be amazed at what is revealed. These kinds of videos can be used to illustrate what was heretofore always imagined. The video can be accompanied by or used in a traditional method of explaining the process of how action potentials are formed.

On April 10, 2019, the first photograph of a black hole or singularity was revealed to the public. Einstein had predicted this in a paper of his that was published in 1915 (Flam, 2019, April 11). Now, 104 years later, the first photograph of a black hole has been made. Black holes, or singularities, are now proven to exist, thanks to technology and clever scientists who know how to use it. How amazing this is!

Literature

The study of literature has been enhanced by new and improved technology. Imaging technology makes it possible to capture the fading documents and manuscripts and restore the images to their original beauty. These images are stored on servers in various world-famous museums. For example, the *Book of Kells* in Ireland is available via imaging technology. This ancient book dates from about the year 800 AD. Our own papers of state, including the original Declaration of Independence, has been restored using both old and new technology. The original works of Shakespeare and other notable authors have been rejuvenated by technology. Many of the classic works of literature are available online and are free to use since their copyright dates have long since expired. These digitized versions are excellent for input into various text analysis applications that make it relatively easy to conduct word frequency studies and other kinds of analyses.

Such technology is especially useful for recording and analyzing folk tales and old ballads as a form of serious literature. The writings of some of America's most famous authors such as Washington Irving, Nathaniel Hawthorne, Edgar Allen Poe, and others have folk tale qualities. The world is forever indebted to Joel Chandler Harris and his collection of Uncle Remus stories. These stories are essentially archetypes of similar tales from other cultures and countries.

Digitizing technology again comes to the aid of the folklorists. The Smithsonian contains many early recordings of folk musicians who performed songs from as far back in time as the middle ages and from Scotland, Ireland, and England to the Appalachian region of the Southern United States. The movie, *The Song Catcher*, tells the story of one of the early folklorists who captured these ballads in the Southern Appalachian region. These unique and essentially priceless artifacts can be put in digital form and thereby preserve them from the wear and tear of use by students of such material and thus made available for the use of scholars of the future. Though it is increasingly difficult to find those who are in a direct line with the bards of the past, digital recorders with sensitive microphones, as well as other capabilities that are built into mobile telephones, make it easy to capture such material. This is a direct entre to oral histories. These personal reminiscences are easy to capture on cell phones and more sophisticated digital recording devices. Once captured they can be studied and analyzed. The information explosion is highly dependent upon existing and emerging technology. The information captured, stored, and circulated by these devices can be turned into knowledge by current and future scholars.

Archaeology

Advances in technology have been of significant benefit to archaeologists. Such advances have moved the archaeologist from extensive work in the field to the computer console. It is now a common practice to scout potential locations of ancient cities and dwellings through satellite images. For example, Google Earth has become a resource for this kind of activity. The images of the earth captured and presented by Google Earth can reveal traces of ancient activity to the observant archaeologist. For example, according to "Archaeologist Uses Satellite to Find Viking Settlement Deep into N America" (n.d.)

Sara Parcak used pictures taken by satellites over four hundred miles above the Earth to seek out indications that Vikings ventured many miles more into North America than previously believed. Parcak had previously used this modern technique to find 17 pyramids, 1,000 tombs, and 3,000 lost civilizations. However [sic] this newest discovery might change everything we have previously "known" regarding Vikings in North America (para. 2).

Light detection and ranging (LIDAR) is another tool that archaeologists use. This technology is applied from airplanes that fly over the area being mapped. LIDAR allows the archaeologist to strip away jungle cover, for example, to find cities that are covered by the vegetation. Ground-penetrating radar is another example of technology used for exploration. The searcher simply moves this device over the ground, and it reveals signs of structures beneath the earth. Archaeologists use endoscopic like devices inserted through holes to peer inside sites that may warrant excavation. Similarly, they can use small mobile robots carrying cameras to explore through wider openings.

Side-scan sonar is becoming more and more vital to archaeological research conducted underwater. This device renders startlingly clear images of structures and debris far beneath the surface of the ocean or landlocked lakes. Similar instrumentation is finding use in monitoring underwater and archaeological heritage sites. This is just some of the technology that archaeologists use in their exploration expeditions. These non-invasive devices can more easily identify areas worthy of excavation, thus saving time and money.

SUMMARY

The information explosion is real. It became obvious beginning in the 1900s. While information is being generated at an exponential rate, our ability to process it remains relatively constant. The issue becomes one of learning to make the most of the limited capacity to intake, analyze, and apply this rapidly growing knowledge more efficiently and effectively. Artificial Intelligence offers a way to screen this mass of data to help scholars and interested others to address the problem of dealing with such a mass of data. A way to achieve this end is through instructional technology and developing a different attitude and approach to learning. A new conceptual approach offers some promise to meet this challenge.

Chapter 2 is an exploration of how we know about the world external to our bodies. What we know is what is perceived by our senses. This discussion leads to an examination of how the brain works and how memories are formed, stored, and retrieved. Memory is affected by emotions, nutrition, and other factors. Next is examined neuroplasticity and neurogenesis along with cognitive load and ability of schemata to compensate for our ability to store and retrieve information lodged in our memories. This is followed by how SMART technologies can enhance our ability to learn and to remember.

REFERENCES

Archaeologist uses satellite to find Viking Settlement deep Into N America. (2016). Retrieved from https://sputniknews.com/us/201604031037419801-archaelogist-uses-satellite-find-viking-settlment-deep-into-north-america/

Civil War Casualties. (n.d.). Retrieved from https://www.battlefields.org/learn/articles/civil-war-casualties

David, L. (2017). *Learning theories in plain English.* Retrieved from https://www.learning-theories.com/

Despopoulos, A., & Silbernagle, S. (1983). *Color atlas of physiology* (2nd ed.). New York: Thieme, Inc.

Drucker, P. F. (1998). *The next information revolution.* Retrieved from http://www.s-jtech.com/Peter%20Drucker%20-%20the%20Next%20Information%20Revolution.pdf

Encyclopaedia Britannica. (n.d.). *William Caxton: English printer, translator, and publisher.* Retrieved from https://www.britannica.com/biography/William-Caxton

Lundell, P. (2014, March 4). *The knowledge doubling curve.* Retrieved from https://www.peterlundell.com/the-knowledge-doubling-curve/

The Smithsonian. (2018). *Timelines of history: the ultimate visual guide to the events that shaped the world* (2nd ed.). New York: DK.

Chapter 2
How We Know the External World

ABSTRACT

The quest begins by examining the means by which the external world is made known. These data are acquired by way of the senses. In the process, these light, mechanical, and chemical inputs are transduced into electrical impulses and routed to appropriate areas of the brain. Our brain translates these data into conscious impressions. These impressions are routed to our memory, which is divided into sensory, short-term, working, and long-term memory. The retrieval process is the reverse of the storage process. The brain can rewire (neuroplasticity) itself to overcome deficits caused by traumatic injury. Cognitive load, which is limited, can be increased by the formation of schemata. SMART instructional technologies can do much to enhance learning, memory formation, and retrieval.

HOW WE KNOW THE EXTERNAL WORLD

Learning implies that one must have data about the outside world about which one arrives at knowledge. The source of these data is our five senses: taste, touch, smell, sight, and sound. Yet, one must consider Hellen Keller who was both blind and deaf from her infancy and therefore deprived of two of the most useful channels of communication with the outside world. Even so, once her teacher, Anne Sullivan, was able to break through the barriers caused by the absence of Ms. Keller's sight and sound perception, her mental

DOI: 10.4018/978-1-7998-1542-6.ch002

Figure 1.

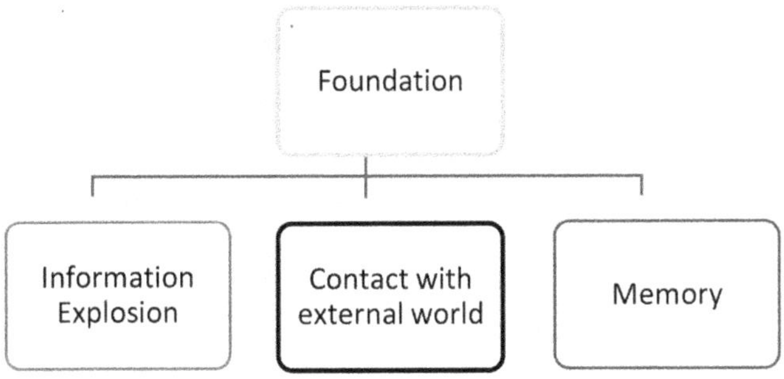

powers were such that she became an influential author, lecturer, and activist ("Interesting Facts About Helen Keller", n.d.). This phenomenon shown by Ms. Keller reveals that one can function at a high intellectual level based on the remaining senses of touch, taste, and smell. One's brain can still make sense of the world. In short, learning can occur, even without functioning five senses, a limitation need not cause one to fail to learn.

Where does this learning take place? It takes place in the brain, which houses the mind. Now arises the question: How? The short answer is that no one really knows, but the answer is becoming nearer and clearer. For example, trial and error taught humanity many things about the process of learning: the role of practice, the role of getting new knowledge based on what is already known, the role of behaviorist conditioning, the role of constructionism, and a host of other theories. These theories (more than 100 of them) (David, 2017) are, for the most part, based on anecdotal evidence derived from observation, deep thought, and formal studies.

The growing knowledge of the brain's physiology is revealing more and more of the secrets of how the brain and the mind work. There are two opposing views of the relationship between the mind and the brain. Those who maintain that the mind is invisible, and the brain is an organ are considered dualists. The dualist view is captured in a metaphor of the computer: The computer is analogous to the brain; the software is analogous to the mind (Barnwal, 2018). Those who maintain that the mind and the brain are the same are considered materialists (Sage, 2011).

HOW THE BRAIN WORKS

It is beyond the scope of this book to delve too deeply into the physiology of how the brain works, but it does bear a superficial examination. Communication with the outside world is obtained via the five senses: sight, sound, touch, taste, smell. These various mechanical and chemical inputs are translated (transduced) into electrical impulses. Sight, for example, is the result of the images of light that is focused by the lens upon the retina. The rods and cones in the retina receive these stimuli and convert them to electrical impulses (Despopoulos & Silbernagle, 1983, p. 301). These impulses are transmitted via the optical nerve to the thalamus where they are sorted and routed to the visual cortex where these impulses are converted into what is seen as pictures and are transmitted to the amygdala which decides if there is an emergency. If there is an emergency, the amygdala recruits other areas of the brain with appropriate speed and relevance. The next stop, in non-emergency situations, for additional evaluation is the hippocampus. The information is held there for a time. Over that time, the hippocampus organizes, distributes, and shuttles these findings to the cortex for long term storage where they become memories (Preston & Echenbaum, 2013). High bias content (that which is considered of great importance) is more likely to be saved rather than low bias content (that which is considered of lesser importance).

SHORT TERM AND LONG-TERM MEMORY

These considerations lead to the phenomena of short-term and long-term memory. One significant element in the act of learning is memory and the ability to recall information as needed from that memory. This operates along the lines depicted in Figure 2. We are bombarded by information or stimuli from the outside world at a rate of approximately 1,000,000,000 (one billion) bits per second (Despopoulos, A., & Silbernagle, S., 1983). This is called sensory memory and has a large capacity and a short duration of between one half a second to two seconds. Then, something grabs our attention and is passed on to working memory. Working memory has a short-term capacity that can handle nine (plus or minus two) chunks of information (Miller, 1994) and is of a short duration of 15 to 20 seconds. This information is either forgotten or moved into long term memory. Long term memory has a very greatly expanded capacity that can retain information indefinitely.

Long term memory is, however, subject to interference, which can inhibit the recall process.

Then something triggers the memory and sets into motion the retrieval process. The sought-after memory is retrieved, processed, moved into working memory, and then moved to our consciousness. The weakest link is the retrieval process from long term memory.

Figure 2 represents how humans process information. For example, stimuli from the outside world impinge on sensory memory. These data are either ignored and routed to forgetfulness or sent on to working memory. From sensory memory, the stimuli that get the attention is routed to working memory. If the message lacks significance, it is routed to forgetfulness. If it is deemed important it is routed to long term memory where it is stored, perhaps indefinitely. When one's memory is triggered, the sought-after memory is retrieved from long term memory, routed to working memory, and then to consciousness. The key to this process lies in triggering and retrieving that information that has been remembered.

Memories incorporate the impressions received from the external world. These include all the five senses: vision, hearing, taste, smell, and touch, as well as emotion. Consequently, these all-encompassing memories seem to be stored in different areas of the brain. The memory coordinates, retrieves, and combines these different components of memory into one unit. Consequently, some (Franklin & Mewhort, 2015) view memory as a hologram, with bits and pieces stored in different places, rather than having it stored in one location.

Figure 2. A Simplified Human Information Processing Model

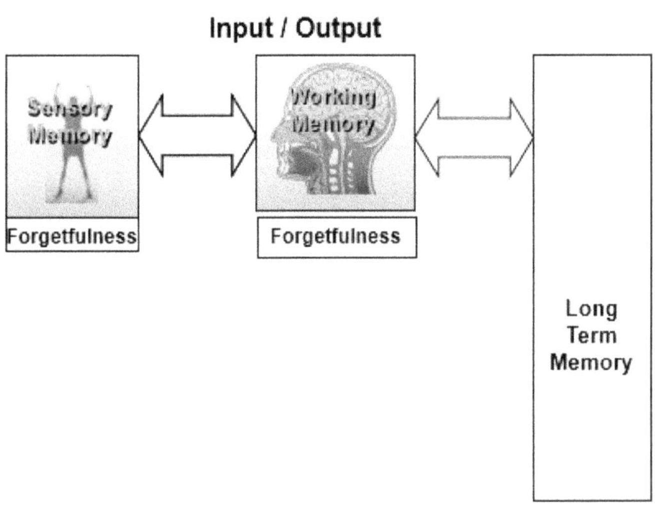

Among many unique qualities, the hologram is such that "… if you break a hologram into tiny pieces, you can still see the entire object in any of the pieces: smash a glass hologram of a cup into bits and you can still see the entire cup in any of the bits!" (Woodford, 2018, How holograms work, para 3).

THE ROLE OF THE EMOTIONS

Emotions play a significant role in what has been remembered, what has been endured over time, and the retrieval of that memory. Concerning instruction, the issue becomes one of how to evoke emotions to promote learning. Perhaps the easiest and least intrusive way is through music. Further, there appears to be a strong association between musical ability and command of language (Jäncke, 2008). It is possible to facilitate learning by use of various forms of music through its ability to stimulate emotions, to encourage dance, and to invoke all three of our domains of knowledge (cognitive, kinesthetic, and affective). However, there are so many variations of musical taste that what may work for one individual may not work for others. Nevertheless, certain principles concern emotional responses to music. For example, a minor key in a slow tempo can invoke a sense of sadness or similar emotions (Hunter, Schellenberg, & Schimmack, 2010). For example, consider Albinoni's Adagio, or Bach's Aire on a G String. A major key in an upbeat tempo, on the other hand, helps to create a sense of happiness and well-being. An example would be one of the marches by John Phillip Souza.

Another finding was that "… women were better at recognizing the emotional pictures than the neutral ones" (Hitti, 2005, para. 4). There are gender-based differences in the ability to perceive emotional states or cues. Brain scans identified the active areas in the amygdala and hippocampus during the identification of the photographs. This region of the brain plays a significant role in emotional memory: its storage and retrieval (Hitti, 2005).

NEUROPLASTICITY

The brain can rewire itself. This is most evident in cases where serious incidents that affected the brain and caused loss of various bodily functions, such as strokes, are often recovered over time. In such cases, the neurons (brain cells) find alternate paths to make new connections that to a degree strive to resolve the deficit. This ability is called neuroplasticity. A group of researchers at the University of Alabama in Birmingham "...found that the combination of neurogenesis and neuroplasticity caused less-fit older neurons to fade into oblivion and die off as the sprightly, young newborn neurons took over existing neural circuits by making more robust synaptic connections" (Bergland, 2017, para. 3). These researchers noted that

Neurogenesis, the creation of new brain cells called neurons, occurs primarily before birth. However, a region of the brain called the dentate gyrus, which is involved in memory, continues to produce new neurons throughout life. Recent studies suggest that adding neurons to the dentate gyrus helps the brain to distinguish between similar sights, sounds, and smells. This in turn makes it easier to encode similar experiences as distinct memories. (Adlaf et al., 2017, p. 2)

As Bergland (2017) noted, the newly formed nerve cells generated by neurogenesis could insinuate themselves into already existing neural networks and perhaps create new memories and may be able to modify older memories. The ability to modify older memories could be of potential value in the treatment of individuals with post-traumatic stress disorder (PTSD).

COGNITIVE LOAD

The working memory of humans is limited in its capacity to process data obtained through the five senses. This leads to the question: How does the brain handle all these sensory inputs? Several researchers, among them Dr. John Swiller, devised the cognitive load theory (Sweller et al. 1998). This theory rests on the caveat that short term memory can hold only seven bits, plus or minus two bits of information (Miller, 1994). Further, cognitive load theory "...aims to understand how the cognitive load produced by learning tasks can impede students' ability to process new information and to create long-term memories" ("Cognitive Load Theory"(n.d.). Even more specifically

Cognitive load is typically increased when unnecessary demands are imposed on a learner, making the task of processing information overly complex. Such demands include the unnecessary distractions of a classroom and inadequate methods used by teachers to educate students about a subject. When cognitive load is managed well, students are able to learn new skills easier than when high cognitive load interferes with the creation of new memories. ("Cognitive Load Theory", n.d.)

Most of us have experienced the effects of cognitive overload. For example, consider the process of scrolling down a webpage and forgetting what one was looking for in the first place. This is but one example of the many things that impinge upon thinking and concentration when engaged in an intellectual or cognitive task. The wise teacher or designer must always remember the effects of cognitive overload and try to minimize it.

SCHEMATA

Schemata consist of anything that one has learned, and each exists as single units in long-term memory. Of the three types of cognitive load (intrinsic, extraneous, and germane), germane concerns the formation of schemata. A schema is a conceptualization of a process or situation or objects. A schema can consist of any number of elements that make up a whole. This schema then combines elements into a single unit in the seven, plus or minus two, capacity that working memory can effectively handle. Teachers should take steps to promote the formation of schemas.

One might wonder how we addressed these issues in times past before there was any direct knowledge of how the brain processed sensory input, formed schemata, stored in long term memory, and retrieved this knowledge as needed. To address these issues, various scholars derived theories of learning that were, for the most part, developed from observation and anecdotal evidence. As it turns out, what has been discovered about how the brain works to support these theories to varying degrees. There are, however, a host of theories that focus on one or a few aspects of learning.

There are similar discoveries that led to the emerging and growing phenomenon called brain-based learning or teaching. Brain-based learning confirms various assertions made by numerous learning theories. Many of these assumptions and assertions are being confirmed by science. Regardless of the learning theory or theories that one may use, consideration must be made of how to appeal to the varied capacities of the brain. Table 1 contains the necessities of Smart technology to take advantage of the current understanding of how the brain works. The two primary senses addressed are sight and sound. Taken separately, our hearing can handle about seven bits per second, while vision can accommodate about 50 bits per second.

Hearing and seeing simultaneously expands to a vast capacity of approximately one million (1,000,000) bits per second, which is a remarkable increase in capability (Despopoulos & Silbernagle, 1983). Adding additional sensory inputs (i.e. touch, taste, and smell) has not been explored, probably owing to the difficulty of connecting them directly to learning.

Human sensory capabilities are very limited; much falls below and extends above what humans can perceive. For example, we can only see within a narrow range of light waves. Infrared and ultraviolet and the remainder of the entire electromagnetic spectrum are insensible to us. We have had some success in expanding these horizons through microscopes, telescopes, radio, television, and other ingenious devices.

Instant feedback is of considerable importance in the act of learning. This permits immediate adjustments to one's thinking or actions to correct errors. It reduces the learning of inaccurate things that over time become more difficult to unlearn. Without feedback, learning would likely not be possible. Recall learning how to ride a bicycle. Initial mistakes were corrected immediately. As these early mistakes were corrected the ability to ride the bicycle with varying degrees of grace and style were developed. Though this is a psychomotor skill, a similar role is played by feedback in the cognitive and affective domains of learning.

SMART TECHNOLOGIES

SMART technologies are to be used to appeal to more than one sense. The most common senses appealed to are sound and sight. Remember, Despopoulos & Silbernagle (1983) noted that hearing amounted to seven bits per second, vision can handle 50 bits per second, and sound and sight together can handle up to 1,000,000 bits per second. Ideally, online or computer-assisted instructional material can exploit the ability to hear and see through simultaneous and closely synchronized hearing and seeing. Also, immediate feedback on student performance makes a great contribution to learning. Most authoring programs allow designers to build in feedback based on student actions. See Table 1 for more information on the capabilities that SMART technologies should be able to provide.

SMART technologies can accommodate these requirements. According to IGI Global (2015), these

Table 1. Smart technology necessities

Technical Ability	Example	Resource
1. Read	The ability to send and receive text is a valuable activity and should be supported.	Because the text is so important, word processing programs, email programs, and similar software answer this need.
2. Hear	Audio capability is vital to instruction; ranging from an informal lecture to music performance.	Most computers and hand-held devices have reasonably good sound systems, particularly when using a headset.
3. See	Video capability can be most useful for teaching and learning.	Most computers and hand-held devices can transmit and receive visual images in color.
4. Hear and See	Seeing and hearing synchronized images and sounds.	Most computers and hand-held devices can transmit and receive moving images and synchronized sound.
5. Feedback	Immediate feedback is very important for learning to occur. This feedback can be accomplished via various authoring programs to permit interaction with the computer either on-site or online.	This inclusion of immediate feedback requires more sophisticated software (authoring programs) and some skill as an instructional designer to create. There are scores of programs that make authoring multi-media programs easy.

... technologies (include physical and logical applications in all formats) that are capable to adapt automatically and modify behavior to fit environment, senses things with technology sensors, this [sic] providing data to analyze and infer from, drawing conclusions from rules. It also is capable of learning that is using experience to improve performance, anticipating, thinking and reasoning about what to do next, with the ability to self-generate and self-sustain (Key Terms in this Chapter, para. 2).

ADMINISTRATIVE CHARACTERISTICS

Successful applications of SMART technology in the classroom or online also depends upon wise administrative support and maintenance. Institutional administration plays an important role in encouraging and maintaining success in online learning. See Table 2 for some of the ways in which administration can play a powerful role in the online learning environment. The process begins with affective engagement, which is defined by IGI Global (2015) as "Students' positive and negative reactions and feeling toward the curriculum, instructor, and peer(s), including interest, boredom, happiness, sadness, anxiety, like, dislike, feeling of belonging, valuing of learning, appreciation of success in school, and so on" (para. 1).

The administration must make a special effort to know the characteristics of their students. This would involve finding the answers to such questions as those that follow: Are they first-generation college students? To what socio-economic group do they belong? Do they know how to use computers to communicate on the Internet, participate in classes, operate formal programs such as Word, Excel, PowerPoint? What are their ages? Their ethnicity? Their race? In short, make sure that administrators have a clear idea of whom they will serve. These considerations will help decide the pedagogical approach to be used.

Try to match instructional methods to learning styles. Even though the role of learning styles has been diminished or challenged in recent years, it remains helpful to determine which of the three learning styles (visual, kinesthetic, or affective) are most common in one's student population. This will help one to determine how to best address these styles through appropriate instructional strategies, methods, and activities. These considerations should also include evaluation methods other than the written word. For example, visual forms of evaluation could work for those students who are primarily visually oriented. Accommodations could be made for those who are oriented toward hearing. Already, the accommodations movement is making these possibilities more practical. An example of this is the need to include closed captioning in visual media.

Another key element to generating student success is keeping them engaged in the learning process: to motivate them. One of the key elements of engagement is based on teacher behavior in a course. A smile, gentle encouragement, a non-verbal demonstration of acceptance and acknowledgment of a student can strongly promote student interest in a course. More on this is covered in the chapter on Learning Theories.

Administrators would be wise to promote the development of self-efficacy in their students, both in the class and particularly online. Simply put, self-efficacy is helping students to believe in themselves. Kirk (n.d.) notes that "Self-efficacy is commonly defined as the belief in one's capabilities to achieve a goal or an outcome" (para. 1). Self-efficacy can be promoted in at least four ways: 1) mastery experiences, 2) vicarious experience, 3) verbal persuasion, and 4) emotional state.

The key to promote mastery experiences is to set the difficulty of learning exercises and events at a level that is neither too difficult nor too easy. The objective is to set conditions so that the student can accomplish the task and thereby build self-confidence and the willingness to continue with their learning. Students also build confidence by watching others perform a task or do well in class. The response of the observer might be something like "That doesn't seem so hard. I can do it too." Teachers can offer verbal persuasion through encouragement, gentle urging, and otherwise being both helpful and approachable. Positive emotions play a powerful role in learning. Teachers through their behavior, both overt and covert, can contribute greatly to a positive emotional climate.

This process of self-regulated learning "... requires students to independently plan, monitor, and assess their learning. However, few students naturally do this well." (Zumbrunn et al., 2011. p. 3). To do this effectively, students must be motivated. Further, students who are effective self-regulated learners must set goals, plan, possess self-motivation, control their attention, use flexible learning strategies, self-monitor, engage in self-seeking actions, and engage in self-evaluation (Zumbrunn et al. 2011). Fortunately, these skills can be taught either directly or through observation by the student of others who have developed content expertise. For this to be successful, the learner must be motivated to learn and use these skills. For administrative characteristics see Table 2.

MOTIVATION

An additional consideration is the role of student motivation. Table 3 lists some of the necessary components for this realm. Simply having an awareness of how motivation can be engendered can be of considerable importance. Curiosity is closely associated with motivation. A professor or facilitator can

Table 2. Administrative characteristics affecting student success in online learning

Characteristic(s)	Purpose
Affective learning engagement	The administration should initiate and support learning engagement by the student.
Address and recognize essential learner characteristics	Make a successful effort to know the characteristics of your students.
Learning styles	Pay reasonable attention to the learning styles of the various students.
Motivational elements	Consider and invoke motivational factors in online learning environments.
Consider the role of self-efficacy	Consider and use the role of self-efficacy in online classes because online study depends heavily on this variable.
Promote self-regulatory learning skills	Promote self-regulatory learning skills because students who find themselves in the relatively isolated milieu of online courses must become responsible for their own learning.

engender a spirit of motivation by engaging in these activities: 1) build in opportunities for special social interaction among students in the course; 2) make available an audience for student work; 3) situate the academic effort between too easy and too difficult; 4) set academic requirements to reflect real-world situations; 5) offer students meaningful choice when possible; 6) make learning a fun event (The "Encouraging Student Academic Motivation" (n.d.) website). See Table 3 for motivational characteristics.

EXAMPLES

History

History is a story of the past; how and why events came about. People not having knowledge of their history have a form of cultural Alzheimer's disease leaving them without any memories of their past. This is an excellent opportunity to make the subject appealing through engendering interest in the material taught in the course. However, there are those professors who fail to do this, which is unfortunate because their students can develop an antipathy to the subject and thereby miss a rich and vibrant experience of the past.

Table 3. Motivational elements affecting student success in online learning

Characteristic(s)	Purpose
Gender	Female students seem to do better online than do male students.
Age	Though producing mixed results in various studies, it appears that older students participate more in online learning than do younger students.
Student's prior online experience	Though producing mixed results in various studies, a student's previous online experience tended to be a positive indicator of success in subsequent online courses.
Self-determination	Scheutz (as cited in Thorsell, 2014) noted that "The student self-determination theory argues, "community college students who experience a robust sense of belonging, competency, and autonomy will naturally be more engaged" (p. 79).
Social interaction	Thorsell, 2014) noted that "...connecting with others is an emotional experience. Handelsman et al. (as cited in Thorsell, 2014) concluded that emotion is one of the strongest types of student engagement and an important part of intrinsic motivation" (p. 80).
Role of leaders	Several studies (as cited in Thorsell, 2014) "...have shown that transformational leadership style generates deeper engagement in students" (p. 80).
Other factors	Online students demonstrate stronger motivation than on-campus face to face students on three intrinsic motivation scales: to know, to accomplish, and to experience stimulation (Rovai, Ponton, Wighting, and Baker, 2007).

Science

Science attempts and is rather successful in expanding our ability to see and to hear and bring technology to bear upon contemporary life. Science has discovered and given humanity various instruments that permit the expansion of their seeing and hearing. Science has greatly expanded its influence in this current age. In medicine, for example, scientists in that discipline have begun to learn how to treat cancer tailored to the genetics of each person who suffers from this horrible disease. This progress is likely just the beginning of what we can expect as time passes.

Literature

Literature is likely as old as humanity. Consequently, it predates the written word. In preliterate times, the telling of tales and stories and the singing of songs and the recitation of poetry performed several functions: entertainment, instruction, and religious ritual. Now, we have expanded literature to include motion pictures and forms that are different from and yet descended from earlier forms.

Archaeology

The growth of technology has given archaeology an array of new tools with which to search the human past. Archaeologists can now peer down upon the earth from hundreds of miles in space and see the traces of ancient civilizations identifiable through slight variations of color in plant life growing over the site. They can strip away jungle overgrowth and unveil lost cities and lost civilizations hidden beneath the abundant foliage. They can peer beneath the surface of the earth to find disturbances in the soil and undercroft that indicate activity from the distant past. They can also peer beneath the sea and lakes to see what lies under the waters. Archaeology has greatly benefitted from advances in technology that contributes to the information explosion.

As these marvelous inventions come into being, one's brain remains essentially the same. The issue becomes one of making the most of innate abilities to keep pace with ongoing developments. Inroads into this area through instructional and telecommunications technology are taking place. When these technologies are presented in a manner consistent with how the brain operates, ongoing improvement is seen. This will likely bring about a change in how educational institutions function.

SUMMARY

In chapter 2, communication with the external world was discussed. One communicates with the environment through the five senses: sight, sound, taste, touch, and smell. The mechanical and chemical intake via the senses is transformed into electrical impulses. These impulses are routed to appropriate areas of the brain for processing and determining meaning. The brain assembles these electrical impulses into our perception of images, sounds, tastes, smells, and physical sensations all of which elicit appropriate reactions. Emotions play a significant role in how past events are remembered. Further, through neuroplasticity, the brain can rewire itself to compensate for lost ability, for example recovering abilities lost due to stroke or other massive injuries to the brain. Additionally, the brain makes new neurons primarily in the dentate gyrus through a process called neurogenesis. There are at least three kinds of memory: sensory, short term, and long term. The capacity of sensory and short-term memory is limited to seven, plus or minus two chunks of information. The formation of schemata in long term memory compensates for the limited capacity of the other two kinds of memory. Schemata are combined into yet other schemata to produce great memory capacity. SMART instructional technology helps to address the demands of various kinds of sensory input. The most powerful of these combinations is sight and sound. When synchronized they can boost our information input to 1,000,000 bits of information per second. Administrative and motivational considerations can work together to enhance the academic progress of our students.

In chapter three, memory is discussed. How memories are formed, how they are stored, and how they are retrieved. Memories lie at the heart of learning because one must be able to retrieve memories of what he or she has learned. The role of neuroplasticity and neurogenesis receive coverage. Factors that affect memory are covered as are the types of memory. The roles of novelty, chemicals that influence memory, and the function of sleep are explored. The roles of scent, hearing, and vision are discussed. Memory formation and aids to help retrieve information from mnemonics are deliberated. The chapter ends with the necessities of SMART technology and examples from four academic disciplines.

REFERENCES

Adlaf, E. W., Vaden, R. J., Niver, A. J., Manuel, A. F., Onyilo, V. C., Araujo, M. T., & Overstreet-Wadiche, L. (2017). Adult-born neurons modify excitatory synaptic transmission to existing neurons. *eLife*, *6*, e19886. doi:10.7554/eLife.19886 PMID:28135190

Barnwal, M. K. (2018). *Difference Between Mind and Brain*. Retrieved from https://www.techaffair24.com/difference-between-mind-and-brain/

Bergland, C. (2017). *How do neuroplasticity and neurogenesis rewire your brain?* Retrieved from https://www.psychologytoday.com/us/blog/the-athletes-way/201702/how-do-neuroplasticity-and-neurogenesis-rewire-your-brain

Cognitive Load Theory. (n.d.). Retrieved from https://www.psychologistworld.com/memory/cognitive-load-theory

David, L. (2017). *Learning theories in plain English*. Retrieved from https://www.learning-theories.com/

Despopoulos, A., & Silbernagle, S. (1983). *Color atlas of physiology* (2nd ed.). New York: Thieme, Inc.

Encouraging Student Academic Motivation. (n.d.). Retrieved from https://www.interventioncentral.org/behavioral-interventions/motivation/encouraging-student-academic-motivation

Franklin, D. R. J., & Mewhort, D. K. J. (2015, October). Memory as a hologram: An analysis of learning and recall. *Canadian Journal of Experimental Psychology*, *69*(1), 115–135. doi:10.1037/cep0000035 PMID:25730645

Hitti, M. (2005). *Emotions make the memory last*. Retrieved from https://www.webmd.com/balance/news/20050131/emotions-make-memory-last

Hunter, P. G., Schellenberg, E. G., & Schimmack, U. (2010, February). Feelings and perceptions of happiness and sadness induced by music: Similarities, differences, and mixed emotions [Abstract]. *Psychology of Aesthetics, Creativity, and the Arts*, *4*(1), 47–56. doi:10.1037/a0016873

IGI Global. (2015). *Regional development getting smarter with ICT*. Retrieved from https://www.igi-global.com/chapter/regional-development-getting-smarter-with-ict/113111

Interesting Facts about Helen Keller. (n.d.). Retrieved from https://factualfacts.com/interesting-facts-about-helen-keller/

Jäncke, L. (2008, August). Music, memory and emotion. *Journal of Biology, 7*(21), 21.1 - 21.5. doi:10.1186/jbiol82

Miller, G. A. (1994). The magical number seven, plus or minus two: Some limits on our capacity for processing information. *Psychological Review, 101*(2), 343-352. http://dx.doi.org.contentproxy.phoenix.edu/10.1037/0033-295X.101.2.343

Preston, R. H., & Eichenbaum, H. (2013, September). Interplay of hippocampus and prefrontal cortex in memory. *Current Biology*, *23*(17), R764–R773. doi:10.1016/j.cub.2013.05.041 PMID:24028960

Rovai, A. P., Ponton, M. K., Wighting, M. J., & Baker, J. D. (2007). A comparative analysis of student motivation in traditional classroom and E-learning courses. *International Journal on E-Learning*, *6*(3), 413–432. Retrieved from http://search.proquest.com/docview/210329343?accountid=35812

Sage, J. (2011). *Mind, brain and consciousness*. Retrieved from https://www.psychologytoday.com/us/blog/mind-brain-and-consciousness/201101/mind-brain-and-consciousness

Sweller, J., van Merrienboer, J. J. G., & Pass, F. G. W. C. (1998). Cognitive architecture and instructional design. *Educational Psychology Review*, *10*(3), 251–296. doi:10.1023/A:1022193728205

Thorsell, L. A. (2014). Graduate certificates in Ontario colleges: Uniquely engaging in specialized skills development. Higher Education. *Skills and Work-Based Learning*, *5*(1), 74–85. doi:10.1108/HESWBL-08-2014-0037

Woodford, C. (2018). *Holograms*. Retrieved from https://www.explainthatstuff.com/holograms.html

Zumbrunn, S., Tadlock, J., & Roberts, E. D. (2011, October). *Encouraging self-regulated learning in the classroom: A review of the literature*. Metropolitan Educational Research Consortium (MERC). Retrieved from https://scholarscompass.vcu.edu/cgi/viewcontent.cgi?article=1017&context=merc_pubs

Chapter 3
Memory Formation, Storage, and Retrieval

ABSTRACT

The ability to form memories and to retrieve them is fundamental to learning. Neuroplasticity and neurogenesis play a role in this function, as does nutrition, oxygenation, and novelty. There are many types of memory, and the primary of these are sensory, short-term, and long-term. These are further subdivided into yet additional kinds of memory. Perhaps the beginning of memory centers around novelty, which arouses and stimulates the brain, through curiosity. Then, there are many memory pathways. Memories are associated with emotions, scent, hearing, vision, to name those with which we are most familiar. To apply this knowledge to education one must consider mastering study skills. This demands that we make a distinction between learning and memory, for each is dependent upon the other and leads to the use of memory aids. SMART applications must capitalize on the ability of technology to help us to see, to hear, and to obtain feedback.

MEMORY FORMATION, STORAGE, AND RETRIEVAL

The role of memory is quite important in retrieving that which was learned. This being the case, it is wise to explore how memory works so that we can exploit what is currently known about this process to promote learning, to make it easier, and to make it more efficient. One definition of memory is that it is "… the reactivation of a specific group of neurons, formed from

DOI: 10.4018/978-1-7998-1542-6.ch003

Figure 1.

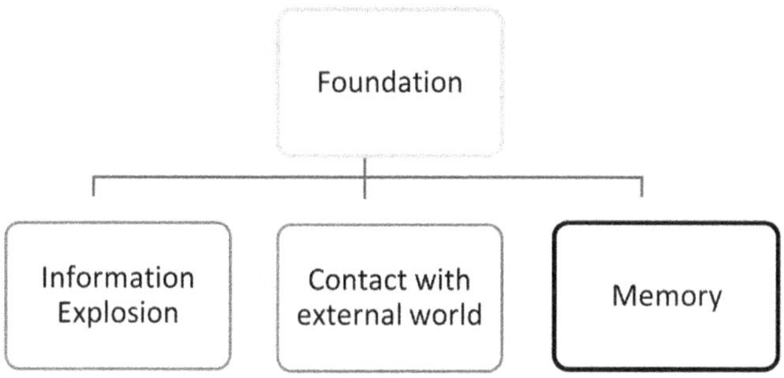

persistent changes in the strength of connections between neurons" (The University of Queensland, 2018, para. 2). This begs the question' How does this happen? The mechanism is termed synaptic plasticity (The University of Queensland, 2018). A synapse is a space between an axon and a dendrite. Upon stimulation, this space becomes flooded with a neurotransmitter that passes the electrical impulse over the gap (synapse) between the transmitting nerve cell to the receiving nerve cell. An increase or decrease in strength is determined by how often these synapses are activated. For example, imagine a grassy lawn. As people walk across this lawn in the same direction, a pathway is worn into the grass. This is like repetitive activity along a neuron, through a synapse, and on to another neuron and another synapse until the impulse reaches its destination. The more this path is used, the stronger the pathway. Yet, synaptic plasticity is perhaps not the only element contributing to the formation of memories. Neurogenesis (the birth of new nerve cells) also affects memory formation. This neurogenesis occurs in the hippocampus. There is some evidence that mice's memory can be improved by increasing neurogenesis. Vigorous physical exercise by humans increases neurogenesis, thereby, likely affecting memory.

Memories form an interconnected assembly of neurons, much like a matrix. This interconnection of neurons is a function of synaptic plasticity. This leads to the realization that memory does not reside in a single location. For example, recall a scene from childhood. Imagine a Sunday afternoon walk with a parent, On one of these walks, they found a hummingbird nest. It was a beautiful and wonderfully made nest of soft fibers. It contained three eggs. That memory resides in not one place but in several. There are the visual images of the nest, the tree branch, the woods, the mellow sunlight filtering through the trees Then, there are sounds associated with the event: the gentle wind whispering through the trees, the sound of the birds, the distant sound of water flowing in the river. There is also a memory of feeling the breeze pass over one's arms, the fresh smell of the forest, the coolness associated with the river. As you can see, this memory involves more than one sense. The various sense memories are stored in different locations in the brain. It is thought that our marvelous brain coordinates the assembly of these sensations and synchronizes them to complete the entire memory.

Emotions play an important role in our memories. Intense emotions like fear or love help memory formation and significance. The University of Queensland Brain Institute (2018) observes that "This happens because of the amygdala, which brain imaging studies have shown is activated by emotional events. ...this boosts memory encoding...by triggering the release of stress hormones, such as adrenaline and cortisol, to boost arousal" (para. 3). Too intense an emotion can have the opposite effect by invoking a more rigid stimulus-response association (The University of Queensland Brain Institute (2018).

NEUROPLASTICITY

Neuroplasticity, According to The Shiel (n.d.) website, is

The brain's ability to reorganize itself by forming new neural connections throughout life. Neuroplasticity allows the neurons (nerve cells) in the brain to compensate for injury and disease and to adjust their activities in response to new situations or to changes in their environment.

Brain reorganization takes place by mechanisms such as "axonal sprouting" in which undamaged axons grow new nerve endings to reconnect neurons whose links were injured or severed. Undamaged axons can also sprout nerve endings and connect with other undamaged nerve cells, forming new neural pathways to accomplish a needed function.

For example, if one hemisphere of the brain is damaged, the intact hemisphere may take over some of its functions. The brain compensates for damage in effect by reorganizing and forming new connections between intact neurons. In order to reconnect, the neurons need to be stimulated through activity (para. 1-3)

Neuroplasticity also includes the process of learning.

NEUROGENESIS

A related phenomenon is neurogenesis. According to the Penguin dictionary of psychology (2009), neurogenesis is defined as the

Growth and development of nerve tissue. In this sense, the term can refer to either the processes involved in the first laying down of neural tissue during gestation and the early phases of development as well as to the growth of new neurons in the mature brain. The latter process was, until recently, thought not to occur and in many texts only the first process will be the intended meaning (para. 1).

One can readily see the connection between neuroplasticity and neurogenesis. The newly formed granule cells develop in the "dentate gyrus region of the hippocampus" (Bergland, 2017). These new granule cells "must become wired into a neural network by forming synapses via neuroplasticity in order to stay alive and participate in ongoing neural circuit function" (Bergland, 2017, para 7). The formation of new nerve cells in mature brains are also theorized to develop in the cerebellum. It is interesting to note that "one of the most effective ways to stimulate neurogenesis and the birth of new granule cells in the hippocampus and the cerebellum" is through physical activity (Bergland, 2017, para. 9). Now, consider factors that affect memory.

FACTORS THAT AFFECT MEMORY

Several factors have an influence on memory. Nutrition is one of them. The memory and cognition of a well-nourished person are generally better than that of a person who is malnourished. Woodhouse and Lamport (2012) note the following:

Given its 100 billion neurons, each with about 2,000 synapses firing around 200 times per second, it is clear that the brain is a bustling place and that cognition is an energy-expensive activity. In fact, the brain accounts for only about 2% of a person's body weight, but consumes between 20-30% of the body's available energy and oxygen (as cited in Woodhouse and Lamport, 2012, p. 5).

The food one consumes affects his or her mood, behavior, and brain function (Fundukian, & Wilson, 2008). Fundunkian and Wilson go on to note that "The human brain is metabolically very active and uses about 20 to 30 percent of a person's energy intake at rest" (para. 5). Instructors must encourage students to eat balanced meals without overindulging or in partaking too little nutrition, and by becoming or remaining physically active.

An allied need to nutrition is adequate oxygenation of the brain. "The brain requires a constant supply of both oxygen and glucose. Without enough oxygen or with low blood-oxygen levels, the brain has trouble signaling where to send blood to oxygen-hungry muscles and tissues" ("Oxygen Levels and Brain Function," 2016, para. 1). Furthermore, the brain consumes about 25% of one's intake of oxygen ("Oxygen Levels And Brain Function," 2016). Rather than passively sitting during instruction, get learners on their feet and moving so that more oxygen will be introduced into their bloodstreams and circulated to their brains.

Novelty plays an important role with respect to influencing our memory. The brain is naturally attracted to anything novel. The area of the brain involved in this response is the substantia nigra/ventral tegmental area (SN/VTA) ("Pure novelty spurs the brain," 2006). Bunzeck and Düzel (2006), whose study was reviewed in the previous sentence, found that humans were driven by stimulus novelty. "Pure novelty spurs the brain," (2006); they also noted that "The SN/VTA exerts a major influence on learning because it is functionally linked to both the hippocampus, which is the brain's learning center, and the amygdala, the center for processing emotional information" (para. 2).

TYPES OF MEMORY

There are several types of memory. The primary forms of memory are three in number: sensory memory that lasts for only about a second, short term memory that lasts for about one minute, and long-term memory that can last for a lifetime. Long term memory can be divided into explicit memory (conscious) and implicit memory (unconscious). Implicit memory is further divided into procedural memory, which amounts to the various skills that we possess. Returning to explicit memory, this can be subdivided into declarative memory, which consists of facts and events. Finally, declarative memory divides into two branches: episodic memory which consists of events and experiences; semantic memory, which is concerned with facts and concepts. See Figure 2.

Cherry (2018b) observed that "Information that you have to consciously work to remember is known as explicit memory, while information that you remember unconsciously and effortlessly is known as implicit memory" (para. 3). For example, explicit memory is that which is involved in consciously memorizing something, something like material for a test in school. Implicit memory is the kind of memory that involves actions that we perform that requires no thought, like the ability to ride a bicycle.

Explicit memory leads to declarative memory, which divides into episodic and semantic memories. Episodic memories are those that recall specific events or episodes in one's life. Examples include what you were doing last week, graduation from school, and so forth. Semantic memory, on the other hand, is of facts, concepts, general knowledge and so on. Implicit memory leads to procedural memory, which refers to the ability to perform automatically certain actions without having to think about them. They are performed unconsciously. Examples include writing with a pen, singing a familiar song, cooking a familiar recipe, and so forth.

Figure 2. The hierarchical arrangement of the types of memory

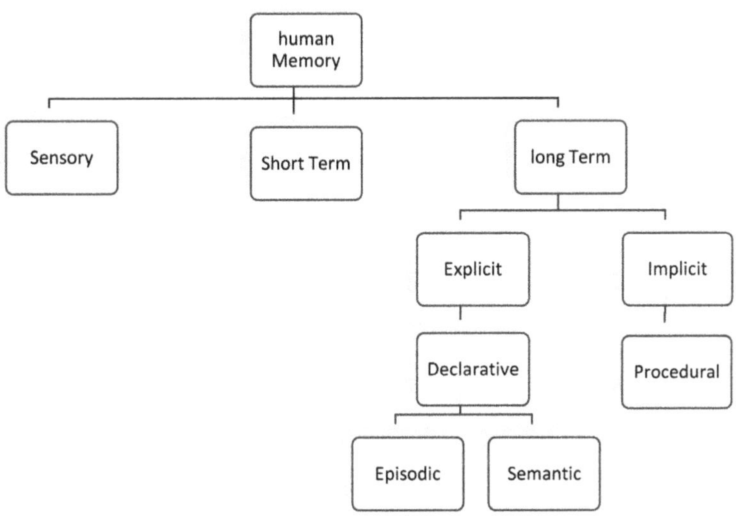

NOVELTY AROUSES A SENSE OF CURIOSITY

With respect to teaching and learning, we can draw from the finding that it would be wise to introduce novelty into instruction so that the minds of students can be drawn into the lesson. Instructional technology offers many opportunities to take advantage of this trait. For example, one can build in images and sounds that are novel to the learner. As Mohs noted (n.d.), "To properly encode a memory, you must first be paying attention" (para. 8). It is significant to note that how we pay attention strongly affects how much we will remember (Mohs, n.d.).

CHEMICALS

The brain performs 100,000 chemical reactions every second that works like a radio transmitting electrical signals (Mehta, n.d.). The brain depends upon several chemicals that help receive and interpret information. These substances are neurotransmitters that facilitate the conduction of electrical signals across the synaptic spaces that separate the axon from the dendrite (Mehta, n.d.). Neurotransmitters form four primary systems: "The dopamine system, noradrenaline system, serotonin system, and cholinergic system are the major neurotransmitter systems in the brain" (Mehta, n.d. para. 2). Depression can also result from serotonin and norepinephrine, and in some cases from dopamine. Conversely, serotonin and acetylcholine can make one happy. Finally, chemical imbalances lead to various problems.

SLEEP

The value of sleep has been recognized for perhaps as long as the human race has existed. Shakespeare recognized the value of sleep as testified to by these lines from Macbeth, Scene 2:

Sleep that knits up the ravell'd sleeve of care,

The death of each day's life, sore labour's bath,

Balm of hurt minds, great nature's second course,

Chief nourisher in life's feast, --

Dr. Mache Seibel (n.d.) notes what happens during sleep "...that the spaces between the brain cells widen and cerebrospinal fluid, the liquid surrounding the brain's cells, floods into these widened spaces during sleep and flushes away the debris" (para. 6). Also, sleep restores the brain as toxic waste is removed from its environment. This knowledge helps teachers recognize the value of sleep and to promote this to their students.

MEMORY PATHWAYS

There are as many memory pathways as there are elements that form memories. Our sensory input is by way of the five senses: sight, sound, smell, touch, taste. Additionally, there are emotions or feelings and movement that provides three-dimensional perspectives, which are spatial in nature (American Geriatrics Society (AGS), Health in Aging Foundation, n.d.). One tends to remember in the context of the first formation of that memory. For example, consider an emotional state associated with a memory. For example, imagine having an intense feeling of joy upon having learned a first complete song on the banjo, *Little Brown Jug*. Conversely, imagine the great sense of sadness when a parent dies. One situation was great joy; the other situation was great melancholy. There are many such memories that are associated with emotions. All of us have had similar experiences.

Scent and Memories

Scent can trigger powerful memories. On a late Spring day in North Carolina, the air was filled with the sweet smell of jasmine. That beautiful plant seemed to grow everywhere with its yellow trumpet-shaped flowers and the enchanting smell of those blossoms. On the other hand, the custom of having flowers at funerals seem to signal sad responses. One might wonder why the sense of smell is so effective in triggering emotions. White (2015), observes that " The olfactory bulb has direct connections to two brain areas that are strongly implicated in emotion and memory: the amygdala and hippocampus. Interestingly, visual, auditory (sound), and tactile (touch) information do not pass through these brain areas." (para. 2). In an experiment using brain imaging that was conducted by Hertz and colleagues, the data revealed via functional magnetic resonance imaging (fMRI) discovered that

When smelling the EO [experimental odor], participants showed the greatest activation in the amygdala and parahippocampal gyrus (a region surrounding the hippocampus). These data suggest that odors that trigger strong, emotional memories also trigger elevated activity in the brain areas strongly linked to emotion and memory (cited in White, 2015, para. 6).

If a memory has an emotional meaning one will be more apt to remember it under similar circumstances (American Geriatrics Society (AGS), Health in Aging Foundation, n.d.).

Hearing and Memory

Another memory pathway is through sound. The sounds can be anything capable of being heard (e.g. the buzzing of a bee, the song of a bird, the growl of an animal, an explosion, a recited poem, etc.). The response to these sounds is entirely personal. For example, consider the sound of fireworks. This may induce a feeling of happiness and excitement in those who have not been in combat. On the other hand, the explosive sounds may trigger a flashback to terrible events for war veterans who have post-traumatic stress disorder. Music is a powerful manipulator of moods. For example, consider the mood induced by the adagio movement in Vivaldi's Concerto in do magg per mandolino, archi e cembalo RV 425 and compare it to the mood induced by the first movement of that same concerto or by the first movement of Khachaturian's *Masquerade Suite*.

Vision and Memory

This is a powerful memory pathway. Imagine seeing a Mocking Bird and hearing its song. Your mood can be changed from a rather joyous reveling in the song of that polyglot bird to one of nostalgia when listening to the music of the song, *Listen to the Mockingbird*, in which the singer tells of this bird singing over the grave of his recently deceased young bride. As noted by American Geriatrics Society (AGS), Health in Aging Foundation (n.d.) "That image is affected by your mood and what you've been thinking about since originally seeing it" (para. 8). As the old bromide goes, "A picture is worth a thousand words." One can invoke visual images to promote memorization by associating a visualization with a relevant situation. For example, consider the following:

Suppose you want to try to remember the decadence of the late Roman emperors such as Caligula and Nero. Try to imagine a banquet with toga-clad people gorging themselves and throwing grapes at one another. That scene will help you remember better than you would if someone just told you to remember the words Caligula, Nero, and decadence (American Geriatrics Society (AGS), Health in Aging Foundation (n.d., para, 9).

Visual Imagery and Memory

Visual imagery is closely associated with one's vocabulary and mastery of language. Combining visual imagery (or other senses) with words for cueing memory is perhaps the most powerful means for memorization. When one uses multiple channels for enhancing memory that memory will be stronger and easier to recall (American Geriatrics Society (AGS), Health in Aging Foundation (n.d.). When compared to adolescents and adults, young children have a greater aptitude for visual memories than they do for word memories. This is a function of vocabulary. One can increase one's ability to remember based on verbal cues by expanding one's vocabulary. This has profound ramifications for instruction and learning.

Study Skills Mastery

What is now known about how the brain operates can help one apply some of these principles to learning. Study skills mastery can include the use of pre-exposure to content, mind mapping concerning the content, application of the stages of optimal learning, the involvement of what one already knows, elaboration of what one learns, and promotion of the formation of memory.

Pre-Exposure

Pre-exposure could be essentially the same as presenting an overview of what is to be learned, thus putting it into a context that makes learning easier. Ausubel's (1960) advanced organizer is a form of pre-exposure. It is a preview of what is to come.

Mind Mapping

According to "What Is Mind Mapping? and How to Get Started Immediately" (n.d.), "A mind map is a graphical way to represent ideas and concepts. It is a visual thinking tool that helps to structure information, helping you to better analyze, comprehend, synthesize, recall and generate new ideas" (para 1). Mind mapping appears to mimic the way human brains operate. It goes beyond linear thinking and is creative. It has the characteristic of novelty to which the brain responds.

Stages of Optimal Learning

Jon Bergmann listed four stages of competence or mastery: unconsciously incompetent, consciously incompetent, consciously competent, and unconsciously competent.

The stages listed in Table 1 need to be explored. The unconsciously incompetent person does not know that he or she does not know. They are in a state of unconscious ignorance. Upon reaching the consciously incompetent state, the learner is aware that he or she does not know. They are no longer completely ignorant. The consciously competent knows that he or she is competent in the task. When the unconsciously competent stage is achieved, he or she is so good at the task that they no longer even consider their competence. Competence is taken for granted.

Four Phases of Learning

Through directed toward training, this model should work well with university students. The model's four phases are preparation, presentation, practice, and performance (Camm, 2011). The key element in the preparation phase is to pique the learner's curiosity and create a positive social environment. The idea is to help learners become interested in learning. In the presentation phase, learners should respond to the content with interest, enjoyment, and multisensory engagement. Practice is the third phase. In this phase, the material

Table 1. The four states of competence (mastery)

Stage	Example
1. Unconsciously incompetent	Has no knowledge of classical Greek
2. Consciously incompetent	Beginning to learn classical Greek
3. Consciously competent	Just passed a final examination in classical Greek
4. Unconsciously competent	Reads classical Greek without conscious awareness

Bergmann (2016)

that is learned should be applied. Performance is the final phase in which learners are given the opportunity to put what they learned into practice.

Presentation

Once one has obtained the attention of his or her students, the content of the instructional sequence can be presented. If one can relate the content to what the students already know, the learning will be easier. Try to introduce novelty to generate interest. A statistic professor was great at this. He had the mannerisms of Jack Benny and was quite witty. It worked because that was almost 30 years ago, and the professor and the material are still vividly remembered. The second statistics course was quite boring. That professor was something of a computer nerd and administered his tests on, by today's standards, antiquated and hard to operate computers.

Practice

Once the initial instructional sequence has been delivered give students an opportunity to practice what they have just learned. The practice need not be overly elaborate. It should provide the student with the chance to reflect on what they have just learned. This purpose was served by homework assignments. If, however, practice can be offered in class while the material is fresh on the minds of the students it will likely be more effective.

Performance

Performance is practice on a broader scale. The learners should be quite competent to demonstrate what they have learned. One memory comes to mind when learning Morse code while in the Navy. The class began slowly and using the typewriter to copy the messages. These typewriters were designed for radio operators because they were in upper case characters. The result was learning Morse code and typing at the same time. It was quite effective.

Learning Through Elaboration

According to Smith and Weinstein (n.d.), elaboration was defined as "… explaining and describing ideas with many details. Elaboration also involves making connections among ideas you are trying to learn and connecting the material to your own experiences, memories, and day-to-day life" (para.2). The essence of this method is captured in the word elaboration. The key is to elaborate via questioning. Ask yourself questions that demand more and more detail. An example from Smith and Weinstein (n.d.) will perhaps shed some light on the nature of the questioning:

Imagine you're studying World War II, and specifically the attack on Pearl Harbor. You could ask yourself, how did this attack happen? On December 7, 1941, the Imperial Japanese Navy attacked the United States Naval Base at Pearl Harbor. The attack included Japanese fighter planes, bombers, and torpedo planes. Why did this happen? The Japanese intended to destroy the United States' Pacific Fleet so that it could not interfere with Japanese operations. Here you could also ask another type of question: What was the result of this historic event? Well, Japanese casualties were light, while they damaged eight U.S. Navy battleships. The Arizona was among those that the Japanese sunk, and was not raised from the shallow water. U.S. aircrafts were also destroyed, and 2,403 Americans were killed (1,178 were injured). Why is this event important? The day after the attack, Roosevelt delivered his Infamy Speech, the United States formally declared war on Japan, and Japanese-Americans were then relocated to internment camps. You could then go on: how did the U.S. enter the war? How did the Pearl Harbor attack lead up to the release of the atomic bomb? How did the war end? And so on. There are so many ways to explain the idea and add details! (para. 8).

Memory Formation

To begin with, it is important to make a distinction between learning and memory: they are two different functions ("The Brain from Top To Bottom", n.d.). Both learning and memory depend heavily upon one another: "Memory is basically nothing more than the record left by a learning process" ("The Brain from Top To Bottom," n.d., para. 4). Learning depends upon memory because what one already knows is stored, probably, in matrices and forms a context to which new knowledge is added. From this, it can be deduced that the more we know the easier it is to attach new knowledge to that which is already known.

Aids to Memory

There have always been techniques to help remember. Mnemonics is one such method. The Pinola (2016) website lists various mnemonic devices to aid memory. These include Acronyms or Expression Mnemonics, music mnemonics, rhyming mnemonics, and the rhyming peg system. One mnemonic common to math and the order of operations is My Dear Aunt Sally, which means multiply, divide, add, and subtract. Another technique is the memory palace. This one goes back to classical Greece and Rome and continues until modern times. To use this, imagine a house, room, etc. with which one is familiar. Take those things to be remembered and put them in places using the imagination. When the memory is needed, simply go back in one's imagination and retrieve the items. Chunking also helps to remember. Chunking simply means lumping things together. It is based on the concept that short-term memory can remember roughly seven pieces of information, plus or minus two, thus producing a range of between five and nine items. Chery (2018) offers four techniques to improve one's memory: practice by way of memorization, look for connections that tie bits of information together, associate bits of information to one another, and incorporate other memory strategies such as mnemonic devices. Rhymes, jingles, and poetry can aid memory. Recall the nursery rhyme:

Thirty days hath September,

April, June, and November;

All the rest have thirty-one,

Excepting February alone,

And that has twenty-eight days clear,

And twenty-nine in each leap year.

The act of writing things with a pen or pencil helps embed memory of the desired material. While typing works, the manual act of writing the information works much better. There are many ways to enhance and improve one's ability to remember. Just imagine how important this was in the olden days before indexing was invented, and books were contained on scrolls. Scholars in those days had to have superb memories.

SMART APPLICATIONS

Now it is time to turn attention to ways to harness what is known about the brain, learning, memory, and retrieval. While the learning mechanisms likely remain the same, access to technology that can make the process of learning more effective and more efficient. This smart technology should have the characteristics depicted in table 2.

The more the technology satisfies all five requirements, the more likely it is to affect rapid learning, memory formation, and retrieval. Evolving communications technology has made it possible to promote and engage in learning anywhere, any time. Learners can take advantage of break time at work, time while waiting, and other snippets of time by using their personal digital devices.

For example, iPads and similar devices have considerable processing capacity. With the emergence of learning management systems that are housed in the cloud, it is possible to use sophisticated applications without the need to house them on our devices. In effect, our devices become an interactive screen for programs housed in the cloud. The only serious drawback concerns the composition of formal papers on these small, keyboardless devices.

Table 2. Smart technology necessities

Technical Ability	Example	Resource
1. Read	The ability to send and receive text is a valuable activity and should be supported.	Because text is so important, word processing programs, email programs, and similar software answer this need.
2. Hear	Audio capability is vital to instruction; ranging from an informal lecture to music performance.	Most computers and hand-held devices have reasonably good sound systems, particularly when using a headset.
3. See	Video capability can be most useful for teaching and learning.	Most computers and hand-held devices can transmit and receive visual images in color.
4. Hear and See	Seeing and hearing synchronized images and sounds.	Most computers and hand-held devices can transmit and receive moving images and synchronized sound.
5. Feedback	Immediate feedback is very important for learning to occur. This feedback can be accomplished via various authoring programs to permit interaction with the computer either on-site or online.	This inclusion of immediate feedback requires more sophisticated software (authoring programs) and some skill as an instructional designer to create. There are scores of programs that make authoring multi-media programs easy.

Connelly & Miller (2018).

EXAMPLES

First, one must have some knowledge of how memories are formed and retrieved. The brain likes novelty. When something new attracts attention, close attention is given to it, at least in the beginning. On the other hand, the brain becomes quickly bored and attention wavers. Emotions can trigger memories if they are like the emotions felt when they were formed. The sense of smell is closely associated with human emotions.

History

Consider how to fix the events of the history example into one's memories. The topic of instruction is the Southern perspective on the War Between the States. This provides an excellent opportunity to generate empathy for the people of the South. The popular music of those times can be used to create emotional states. Descriptions of the depravations created by Sherman's soldiers on their march to the sea may contribute to arousing feelings of empathy. The Rebel Yell can create a strong psychological state of either fear or aggression. Excerpts from books can provide the reasoning of the people of the South concerning the war.

Science

Consider how to fix the events of our science example into memory. Begin by creating a novel situation. For example, video of the electrical impulses generated by calcium signaling in the heart accompanied by sounds of the heartbeat can be a powerful source for forming memories. The skillful repetition of the elements that generate memories can be applied to create "paths in the lawn" in our mind.

Literature

Consider how to fix the events of our literature example into memory. Literature by its very nature is evocative of emotions. The emotions can range from pathos to humor, depending upon the story or song. The motif of folk stories and songs are varied and are typically funny or sad or nonsense. One can use dramatizations of folk stories or have musicians perform folk songs. These will likely capture the attention and imagination of your learners.

Archaeology

Consider how to fix the events of the archaeology example into memory. Dramatization can make a profound introduction to a unit. For example, one could play excerpts from programs about using Google Earth to find traces of ancient civilizations or excepts using side-scan sonar, or LIDAR. These technologies are quite impressive and will likely remain the memories of your student.

SUMMARY

The ability to remember is one of the most human and vital activities. To gain a better understanding, look at how the brain operates and its idiosyncrasies. Neuroplasticity describes the ability of the brain to rewire itself. Neurogenesis describes the lifelong ability of certain areas of the brain to continue to produce nerve cells. There are factors that affect memory. Some of these are nutrition, exercise, oxygenation, and so forth. There are various types of memory, such as sensory, working, short-term, and long-term memory. These are divided into yet other kinds of memory. That which is novel captures attention by invoking a sense of curiosity. The brain is a hotbed of chemical and electrical activity. Sleep is vital to wellbeing. It is thought that during sleep debris in our brain is flushed away, as well as other actions that take place to refresh us. Be aware of memory pathways. The effect of scent, hearing, vision, visual imagery and touch on our memories is profound. Knowing what is known now and what is being learned, one can apply this knowledge to study skills, which brings up the four phases of learning: preparation, presentation, practice, and performance. Elaborate on what is being learned to make it more fun and to help retain it longer. All of this helps form memories. There are effective aids to memory. SMART applications can help retain more of what is learned. Memory is a powerful force.

Chapter 4 has a discussion of various theories of learning in the context of four primary theories (i.e. behaviorism, cognitivism, constructivism, and connectivism). Then the role and nature of instructional objectives are covered. This is followed by consideration of the age of the learner, the nature of the subject, time available for instruction, learner interest with an exhortation to make the instruction interesting.

REFERENCES

American Geriatrics Society (AGS), Health in Aging Foundation. (n.d.). *Memory pathways*. Retrieved from https://www.dummies.com/health/mental-health/memory-pathways/

Ausubel, D. P. (1960). The use of advance organizers in the learning and retention of meaningful verbal material. *Journal of Educational Psychology*, *51*(5), 267–272. doi:10.1037/h0046669

Bergland, C. (2017). *How do neuroplasticity and neurogenesis rewire your brain?* Retrieved from https://www.psychologytoday.com/us/blog/the-athletes-way/201702/how-do-neuroplasticity-and-neurogenesis-rewire-your-brain

Bergmann, J. (2016). *The five stages of mastery learning*. Retrieved from http://www.jonbergmann.com/the-five-stages-of-mastery-learning/

Bunzek, N., & Duzel, E. (2006). Absolute coding of stimulus novelty in the human substantia nigra/VTA. *Neuron*, *3*(51), 369–379. doi:10.1016/j.neuron.2006.06.021 PMID:16880131

Camm, B. (2011). *The four phases of learning*. Retrieved from https://www.dashe.com/blog/instructional-design/four-phases-of-learning/

Cell Press. (2006, August 27). Pure Novelty Spurs the Brain. *ScienceDaily*. Retrieved March 16, 2019 from www.sciencedaily.com/releases/2006/08/060826180547.htm

Cell Press. (2006, August 27). Pure Novelty Spurs the Brain. *ScienceDaily*. Retrieved March 16, 2019 from www.sciencedaily.com/releases/2006/08/060826180547.htm

Cherry, K. (2018b). *Learn to distinguish between implicit and explicit long-term memory*. Retrieved from https://www.verywellmind.com/implicit-and-explicit-memory-2795346

Connelly, J. O., & Miller, P. (2018). Improving learning outcomes for higher education through smart technology. *International Journal of Conceptual Structures and Smart Applications*, *6*(1), 1–17. doi:10.4018/IJCSSA.2018010101

Fundukian, L. J., & Wilson, J. (2008). Nutrition and Mental Health. In *The Gale Encyclopedia of Mental Health* (2nd ed.; Vol. 2, pp. 785-791). Detroit, MI: Gale. Retrieved from http://link.galegroup.com.contentproxy.phoenix.edu/apps/doc/CX2699900294/GVRL?u=uphoenix_uopx&sid=GVRL&xid=f5def220

Mehta, S. (n.d.). *Chemicals in the human brain and their functions*. Retrieved from https://bodytomy.com/chemicals-in-brain

Mohs, R. C. (n.d.). *How human memory works*. Retrieved from https://science.howstuffworks.com/life/inside-the-mind/human-brain/human-memory1.htm

(2009). Neurogenesis. InReber, A. S., Allen, R., & Reber, E. S. (Eds.), *The Penguin dictionary of psychology* (4th ed.). London, UK: Penguin. Retrieved from https://search-credoreference-com.contentproxy.phoenix.edu/content/entry/penguinpsyc/neurogenesis/0

Nutrition and Mental Health. (2008). In L. J. Fundukian & J. Wilson (Eds.), *The Gale Encyclopedia of Mental Health* (2nd ed.; Vol. 2, pp. 785–791). Detroit, MI: Gale. Retrieved from http://link.galegroup.com.contentproxy.phoenix.edu/apps/doc/CX2699900294/GVRL?u=uphoenix_uopx&sid=GVRL&xid=f5def220

Oxygen levels and brain function. (2016). Retrieved from https://lunginstitute.com/blog/oxygen-levels-brain-function/

Pinola, M. (2016). *The science of memory: Top 10 proven Techniques to remember more and learn faster.* Retrieved from https://zapier.com/blog/better-memory/

Seibel, M. (n.d.). *Sleep does knit the raveled sleeve of care*. Retrieved from https://drmache.com/sleep-does-knit-the-raveled-sleeve-of-care/

Shiel, W. C. (n.d.). *Medical definition of neuroplasticity*. Retrieved from https://www.medicinenet.com/script/main/art.asp?articlekey=40362

Smith, M., & Weinstein, Y. (n.d.). *Learn how to study using... elaboration*. Retrieved from http://www.learningscientists.org/blog/2016/7/7-1

The Brain From Top to Bottom. (n.d.). Retrieved from http://thebrain.mcgill.ca/flash/d/d_07/d_07_p/d_07_p_tra/d_07_p_tra.html#1

The University of Queensland Brain Institute. (2018). *How are memories formed?* Retrieved from https://qbi.uq.edu.au/brain-basics/memory/how-are-memories-formed

What is mind mapping? (and How to get started immediately) (n.d.). Retrieved from https://litemind.com/what-is-mind-mapping/

White, A. (2015). *Smells ring bells: How smell triggers memories and emotions*. Retrieved from https://www.psychologytoday.com/us/blog/brain-babble/201501/smells-ring-bells-how-smell-triggers-memories-and-emotions

Woodhouse, A., & Lamport, M. A. (2012). The Relationship of Food and Academic Performance: A Preliminary Examination of the Factors of Nutritional Neuroscience, Malnutrition, and Diet Adequacy. *Christian Perspectives in Education, 5*(1). Retrieved from http://digitalcommons.liberty.edu/cpe/vol5/iss1/1

Section 2
The Components

Section 2 concerns the various elements or components that can lead to more effective and efficient learning. Chapter 4 contains a discussion of the elements that bear a profound influence on teaching and learning. These influences are the product of various learning theories. These theories supply both a conceptual and theoretical foundation for making learning more effective and efficient. This builds on the contents of Section 1. Over the years, more than 100 learning theories were developed. Of this substantial number of theories, the most popular five of them receive greater attention. These are followed by a discussion of selecting a suitable learning theory to guide development of one's project, the roles of instructional objectives, the age of the learner (maturity), the nature of the subject, the interest of learners in the topic of instruction. Chapter 5 has a discussion of instructional design models. Seven of a greater number of models and theories receive attention. The roles of selecting and applying an instructional design model, the iterative nature of all such models, evaluation of learning, and the feedback are covered next. Chapter 6 contains a focus on the role and characteristics of students, technology, administration, and motivation.

Figure 1.

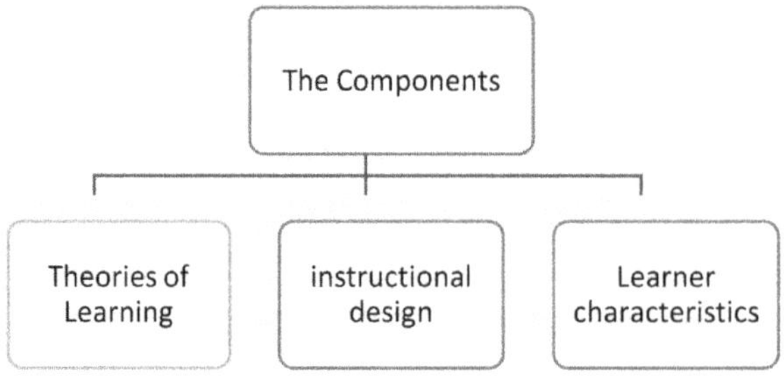

Chapter 4
Theories of Learning

ABSTRACT

There are a host of theories of learning. Many of these have been around for a long while, and all of them offer sound insight into how people learn, but none offer a unifying theory of learning. Of all these theories, four are treated in this chapter: behaviorism, constructivism, cognitivism, and connectivism. The issue becomes one of selecting a learning theory that matches instructional content and learner characteristics. Instructional objectives guide how the instruction is to be delivered and assessed. These objectives cover three domains: cognitive, psychomotor, and affective with skills contained within them structured hierarchically. The learner's age, interests in the subject content, the nature of the subject, and time available for instruction significantly affect the instructional process. The most important thing an instructor can do is to make the content in their course interesting and relevant to their students.

THEORIES OF LEARNING

Over the years approximately 100 theories of learning have been developed and expanded. These theories fit into general classifications: behaviorism, cognitivism, constructivism, motivation and humanist, identity, media and technology, mental models, design theories and models, descriptive and metatheories, child development theories, and paradigms. For a comprehensive list of models, see Appendix A. The more commonly recognized theories are the behaviorist, cognitivist, constructivist, and the connectivist. These four

DOI: 10.4018/978-1-7998-1542-6.ch004

Figure 1.

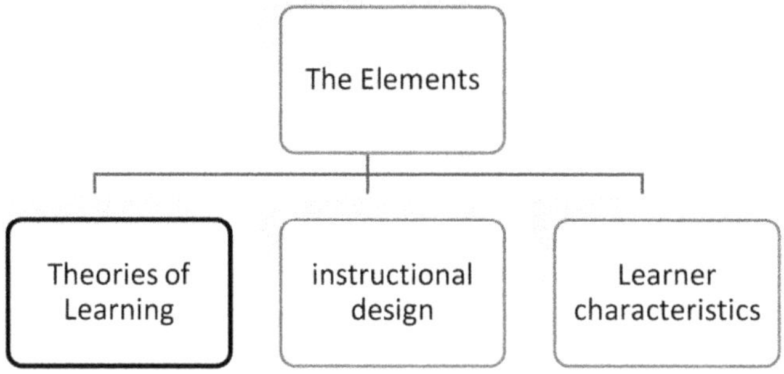

theories were chosen because they are considered by some to be the most popular and appropriate learning theories for online learning ("Learning Theories", 2019; Little, 2015; "Four Top Learning Theories In The Digital Age", 2015). These four are examined in more detail as follows:

BEHAVIORISM

Behaviorism is perhaps the oldest of these four families. David (2017) noted that "Behaviorism is a worldview that operates on a principle of "stimulus-response." All behavior [is] caused by external stimuli (operant conditioning). All behavior can be explained without the need to consider internal mental states or consciousness" (p. 19). A foundational concept holds the view that the learner is a passive vessel who responds to stimuli in his or her environment. Positive or negative reinforcement determines subsequent behavior.

One of the first and most successful examples of the application of behaviorist principles to learning was the military. Faced with the task of training recruits from varied backgrounds and with varied educational attainments, the military chose to use behaviorist principles to prepare these diverse individuals to function in demanding jobs with high degrees of competence. A former petty officer was a product of this training in the Navy in the mid-1960s. He took an aptitude test in boot camp that indicated that he would make a great radioman. Upon being asked if he would like to do this, he strongly agreed. It turned out that he excelled in this rating.

At this sailor's first duty station at a remote radar site in Iceland (H2), he was within a few weeks after arriving there made the transmitter deck supervisor of his watch. At his next duty station onboard the USS Adroit

(MSO-509), he was soon the leading radioman for the division of four ships. A short stint in the CIA as a telecommunications specialist followed next where he worked as the second radioman in a two-man station. He went on to more and more responsible positions onboard a National Oceanographic and Atmospheric Administration (NOAA) research ship as a radio officer. He became an amateur radio operator and still holds his general class license with the call sign N4NGF.

Upon discharge from the Navy, he took a correspondence course (a precursor of distance education before the computer and Internet age) to prepare for the FCC Radiotelephone First Class and the Radiotelegraph Second Class licenses. This correspondence course used what was called programmed instruction, which was based entirely on behaviorist principles. This learning theory really works; he experienced it. It also led to his interest in electronics theory, which constitutes a good part of physics, thus going far beyond the operational objectives of the course.

A more radical form of behaviorism was developed by B. F. Skinner (David, p.20). What contributed to the radical nature of this form of behaviorism was acceptance of the role of emotions and mediating structures. This system of behaviorism seems to be that which drove its application to military training and other forms of training. Skinner also originated the concept of the black box. The black box signifies viewing a system in the context of its inputs and outputs while paying little attention to what happens within the black box. Along with Skinner other contributors to behaviorism were John B. Watson, Ivan Pavlov, E. D. Thorndike, and Albert Bandura (David, p.19).

COGNITIVISM

Cognitivists hold the essential view that the "black box" of the mind should be understood. This theory views the mind as analogous to a computer (David, p. 35). Cognitivism replaced behaviorism in the 1960s as the dominant learning theory (David, 2017). Cognitivism concentrates on the internal world of the mind. "Mental processes such as thinking, memory, knowing, and problem-solving need to be explored. Knowledge is viewed as schemata or symbolic mental constructions. Learning is defined as change in a learner's schemata" (David, 2017, p.35). Unlike the behaviorist view, the cognitivist view holds that humans are not programmed animals but are rational creatures who must actively participate in learning. Sure, humans change their behavior, but this change is due to what is happening in the learner's mind. This learning theory thinks of the mind as a computer in which information is taken, is processed, and is acted upon, thus leading to certain outcomes (David, 2017). Some leading contributors to cognitivism include Marriner David Merill, Charles Reigeluth, Robert Mills Gagne, Jerome Bruner, and Roger Schank (David,2017)

CONSTRUCTIVISM

Constructivists operate on the premise that learning is a constructive, active process in which the learner constructs his or her own knowledge (David, 2017). "Knowledge is constructed based on personal experiences and hypotheses about the environment. Learners continuously test these hypotheses through social negotiation" (David, 2017, p. 1). Consequently, each person creates his or her own interpretation of the knowledge they have acquired. This constructivist theory is subject to considerable confusion. "Constructivism assumes that all knowledge is constructed from the learner's previous knowledge, regardless of how one is taught. Thus, even listening to a lecture involves active attempts to construct new knowledge (David, 2017, p. 41). Those who contributed to this theory include Lev Semyonovich Vygotsky, Jean Piaget, John Dewey, and Jerome Seymour Bruner (David, 2017).

CONNECTIVISM

Connectivism is closely connected to the Internet and is, therefore, a relatively new learning theory. "Connectivism ... explains how Internet technologies have created new opportunities for people to learn and share information across the World Wide Web and among themselves" (David, 2017, p. 39). In other words, these individuals make a connection and learn from one another. These kinds of communication include email, web browsers, wikis, discussion forums, YouTube, and so forth (David, 2017). One element that sets connectivism apart is its insistence that considerable learning takes place in online peer networks (David, 2017). Stated differently, learners cooperate in the learning process and teach and learn from one another in their quest for knowledge.

SOCIO-CULTURALISM

Cherry (2019 July 26), noted that " Sociocultural theory grew from the work of seminal psychologist Lev Vygotsky, who believed that parents, caregivers, peers, and the culture at large were responsible for developing higher order functions" (para. 2). The role of one's cultural milieu in his or her learning and development is of considerable significance in this learning theory. The online culture, then, assumes considerable importance in one's learning; knowledge arises from interaction with other individuals (Cherry, 2019). With respect to online learning, socio-culturalism is similar to connectivism. Application of socio-culturalism in the classroom and online involves an understanding of the zone of proximal development in helping to identify where students are and where they should be and guiding them to expand their zone (Cherry, 2019).

SELECTING A LEARNING THEORY

Remember, these are but four out of roughly 100 learning theories. So, instead of focusing on the individual learning theories, let us give attention to selecting one or more theories that would fit your instructional situation. What criteria would we use to select them? See Table 1 for more information.

The key to the intelligent use of a particular learning theory is to diminish or eliminate personal bias toward any given philosophy of learning. Let the nature of the material and the nature of the learner dictate what theory to use. For example, though having fallen out of favor in recent years, some material responds best to a behaviorist approach because it is a great way to handle fundamental knowledge and ability. Further, some skills (e.g. psychomotor) require considerable practice. For example, becoming a competent shipboard radio operator at, say 20 or more words per minute, requires simple practice. Learning to play a musical instrument requires practice, but this is only the first and the most basic level of musicianship because considerable cognitive knowledge is required as well as affective ability.

Once the fundamentals have been achieved, one can begin to construct his or her knowledge. This construction of knowledge leads one to explore, to mediate, to build, to let the imagination soar while keeping within the limits imposed by the subject matter. The learning content should be governed by the instructional objectives.

Table 1. Criteria for selecting and applying learning theory to an instructional problem

Factors That Affect Instruction	Questions
Objectives of instruction	Would the objectives be more amenable for a behaviorist, cognitivist, constructivist, connectivist, etc. approach?
Age of learner	Are your learners who are very young with little life experience? Are they older and have more life experience? Are they mature adults with considerable life experience?
The nature of the subject	Does the nature of the subject require memorization of fundamentals? Does the subject require lived experience? Is the subject concrete? Is the subject more freewheeling, such as literature?
The time available for instruction	Does the subject require considerable time for instruction? Does the subject require little time for instruction?
The interest of the learner	Is the subject something that interests the learner? Could the learner care less about the material?

INSTRUCTIONAL OBJECTIVES

The purpose of the instructional objective is to provide a foundation upon which to design instruction, organize it, and establish what is to be done, the conditions under which it is performed, and the level of desired competence. For each of three commonly accepted domains, one can compose instructional objectives: cognitive, psychomotor, and affective. A taxonomy of objectives for the cognitive domain was developed by Dr. Benjamin Bloom and his team (Armstrong, 2017). A taxonomy for the affective domain was developed and introduced by Dr. Krathwohl (Bilash, 2011). A taxonomy for the psychomotor domain was developed by Dr. Simpson (Laws, 2015). These taxonomies should clarify and identify behaviors expected of learners after having finished a course of instruction.

Taxonomy is primarily a scientific term that describes a systematic classification of various forms of living organisms. Psychology and other social sciences have broadened the term to include a wider application of taxonomy to include the classification of other variables. The taxonomies are ordered from least complex to most complex. Benjamin Bloom's taxonomy for the cognitive domain illustrates this quite aptly. The lowest skill to the highest skill is knowledge, comprehension, application, analysis, synthesis, and evaluation (Armstrong, 2017). A list of verbs can be compiled for each level of the cognitive domain. See Table 2 for those examples.

Table 2. Action verb examples in Bloom's taxonomy of the cognitive domain

Level	Definition	Verbs	Sample Tasks
Knowledge	Recall previously learned material.	• Arrange • Identify • Memorize • Recognize	• Define the 6 levels of Bloom's taxonomy of the cognitive domain.
Comprehension	Grasp meaning, explain, restate ideas.	Explain Convert Express Infer Rewrite	Explain the purpose of Bloom's taxonomy of the cognitive domain
Application	Use learned material in new situations.	Use Apply Employ Practice Show	Write an instructional objective for each level of Bloom's taxonomy
Analysis	Separate material into component parts and show relationships between parts.	Analyze Change Employ Practice Solve	Compare the cognitive and affective domains
Synthesis	Put together separate ideas to form a new whole, establish new relationships.	Create Design Hypothesize Invent Develop arrange assemble	Design a classification scheme for writing educational objectives that combines the cognitive, affective, and psychomotor domains.
Evaluation	Judge the worth of material against stated criteria.	Judge Recommend Critique Justify Appraise Argue	Judge the effectiveness of writing objectives using Bloom's taxonomy

Adapted from Bixler (n.d.) and http://chiron.valdosta.edu/whuitt/col/cogsys/bloom.html

The affective domain as constructed by Dr. James Krathwohl identifies the levels of affective knowledge. These are, in ascending order, receiving, responding, valuing, organization, and characterization (Bilash, 2011). See Table 3 for examples. The affective domain has to do with the emotions and the feelings of individuals. In some enterprises, this is of vital importance. The musician must be able to interpret a given piece of music, to bring the piece to life, to give it a soul. There are less obvious examples as well. For example, a carpenter must have a feeling for his or her profession. Personal experience with various physicians and surgeons revealed that those who truly loved what they did made a profound difference in their practice of medicine.

Dr. Simpson, the creator of the psychomotor or kinesthetic skills domain, determined that these skills are, in ascending order perception, set, guided

Table 3. Action verb examples in Krathwohl's taxonomy of the affective domain

Level	Definition	Verbs	Sample Tasks
Receiving	Being aware of or attending to something in the environment.	Accept Attend Develop Recognize	Individual reads a book passage about civil rights.
Responding	Showing some new behaviors because of experience.	Explain Convert Express Infer Rewrite	Answers questions about the book, reads another book by the same author, another book about civil rights, etc.
Valuing	Showing some definite involvement or commitment.	Complete Comply Cooperate Discuss Examine Obey Respond	Demonstrates this by voluntarily attending a lecture on civil rights.
Organization	Integrating a new value into one's general set of values, giving it some ranking among one's general priorities.	Codify Discriminate Display Order Organize Systematize Weigh	Arranges a civil rights rally.
Characterization by value	Acting consistently with the new value.	Internalize Verify	Is firmly committed to the value, perhaps becoming a civil rights leader.

Adapted from Bixler (n.d.)

response, mechanism, complex overt response, adaptation, and origination (Laws, 2015). The kinesthetic domain is very important for certain kinds of ability that ranges from simple perception to accomplished adaptation. The psychomotor domain concerns performing physical acts. These acts can range from gross motor skills such as running, lifting heavy objects, and strenuous physical exertion to fine tactile skills such as playing a musical instrument, performing delicate surgery, repairing delicate instruments. See Table 4 for more.

When choosing a learning theory as a conceptual framework, one has many choices among the three domains.

AGE OF THE LEARNER

The age of the learner is very important because there are great differences between the grade school student, the high school student, the university student,

Table 4. Action verb examples in Simpson's taxonomy of the psychomotor domain

Level	Definition	All-Purpose Verbs	Sample Tasks
Observing	Active mental attending of a physical event.	Bend Calibrates Constructs Differentiate (by touch)	Watches a more experienced person. Other mental activities, such as reading may be part of the observation process.
Imitating	Attempted copying of physical behavior.	Dismantles Displays Fastens Fixes Grasp	The first step in learning a skill. The learner is observed and given direction and feedback once. Movement is not automatic or smooth.
Practicing	Trying a specific physical activity over and over.	Grinds Handle Heats Manipulates Measures Mends Mixes Operate	The skill is repeated over and over. The entire sequence is performed repeatedly. Movement is moving towards becoming automatic and smooth.
Adapting	Fine-tuning. Making minor adjustments in the physical activity to perfect it.		The skill is perfected. A mentor or a coach is often needed to provide an outside perspective on how to improve or adjust as needed for the situation.

Adapted from Bixler (n.d.)

and the adult learner. Perhaps this could be shortened to four categories: child, teenager, young adult, and adult. The immature student is addressed through pedagogy; the mature student is addressed through andragogy. The adolescent student can be addressed through both pedagogy and andragogy. The age of the student can have a profound effect on how successful instruction can be. A learner's age can span several variables, including attention. For example, a child has a very short attention span, while the adolescent has a longer one, and the adult has the longest.

THE NATURE OF THE SUBJECT

The nature of the subject must be considered, as well. Is it science? Technology? Engineering? Arts? Math? Then, the diverse aptitudes of our learners must be considered. Some have an aptitude for working with numbers. Others have an aptitude for art, for science, for athletics, and so forth. The complexity of the content must be considered, as well. For example, is rote memory the primary requirement? Does the subject consist of analysis? Is the material entirely new for your learner? Or, is it something that builds on previous knowledge in the subject? As one can see, the nature of the subject becomes a very special area of consideration.

THE TIME AVAILABLE FOR INSTRUCTION

The amount of time available for instruction requires attention. Initially, the attention span of learners must be considered. Children perhaps have the shortest attention span, teenagers have a slightly longer attention span. Adults probably have the longest attention span; however, it must prove to be interesting to all these learners. The professor should make a special effort to match the time available to the brain's need for both novelty and reflection (Jensen, 2008). Too little time spent on a unit of instruction will create difficulties in the future because cognitive knowledge or physical manipulation often builds to progressively more complex activities. Try to match new information or knowledge to that already held by the learner.

THE INTEREST OF THE LEARNER

The degree of interest in the material being taught is another important consideration. If one is interested in the subject, they appear to be more inclined to remember the material and to use it. It is natural for the brain to respond to stimuli that interests it. Jensen (2008) noted that the brain responds well to novelty while requiring time for reflection on that which was learned. The question becomes one of engendering the interest of the learner in the content of the lesson. Luisa Brenton (2016) offers 10 tips on how to accomplish this task:

1. Make it relevant to their everyday lives.
2. Make it enjoyable.
3. Show them the relevance to their future careers.
4. Encourage them to participate in the process.
5. Use multiple instructional resources.
6. Make it personal for them.
7. Defer talking about tests until later.
8. Change the location where the learning takes place.

9. Make the instruction attainable.
10. Relate it to their interests.

Though Brenton slanted this to K-12 students, these tips can easily be applied to students in higher education and adapted to online courses. Generating interest involves making the material relevant to learners' everyday lives and to their future or existing careers. Persons tend to engage in enjoyable activities, so make it enjoyable. Help learners realize the relevance of the material to future careers. Part of the joy and power of learning is participation in the learning process. Use varied instructional technology to appeal to their sensory input. Considerable interest can be generated by making the content personal to the students. Do not destroy the momentum by discussing testing and other housekeeping chores. Plan and conduct field trips and thereby change the location in which learning takes place. Strive to strike a balance between making the material too easy or too difficult, find a middle ground to avoid flagging interest. keep the goals within the learner's reach. Always relate the material to student personal interests where possible.

George Lowenstein (1994) noted that when curiosity is aroused "... attention becomes focused on a gap in one's knowledge. Such information gaps produce a feeling of deprivation, which can be labeled curiosity. The curious individual is motivated to obtain the missing information to reduce or eliminate the feeling of deprivation" ("The psychology of curiosity: A review and reinterpretation," 1994, p. 87). Arising from this theory of information gaps, three steps can stimulate or engender a student's curiosity. Paul (2013) suggests prefacing instruction with a question. The second is quaintly stated as "priming the pump." This action is based on invoking a student's already existing knowledge about the topic. Lowenstein (1994) noted that "...it may be necessary to "prime the pump" to stimulate information acquisition in the initial absence of curiosity" (p.97). The final step is to bring in communication with others about the topic.

Another resource to arouse student curiosity centers around nonverbal teacher behavior. Mazer (2013) explored the influence of teacher behaviors on student engagement and found that students respond positively to certain teacher behaviors. Mazer (2013) observed that an increase in emotional arousal caused by teacher nonverbal immediacy behaviors such as contact, movement, facial expressions, and vocal variety, heightens a student's attention, thus promoting learning.

MAKE IT INTERESTING

No matter what theory one uses, make it interesting and fun. Subjects labeled as boring are not so much boring as they are difficult to relate to owing to lack of visualization or application. Brenton (2016) shares 10 ways to make the subject interesting. This can be done by helping students to see it as a part of their daily lives. Make the topic interesting. Another step would be to try to show how the material could be relevant to their careers. One sure way to reduce boredom would be to encourage participation in the learning event. With the growth of instructional technology, the instructor could divide the class into groups and have them conduct research via WebQuests.

Using multiple resources for instruction could generate considerable interest. Using more than one resource in one's teaching is a good way to generate and maintain interest. For example, illustrating a lecture with a PowerPoint or a similar program can work wonders. Imagine instruction on music. Rather than telling about the structure of a concerto, illustrate one by using a group such as Il Giardino Armonico who performs Baroque music on period instruments. Some of those instruments no longer exist in the cultural mainstream, such as the archlute or theorbo. Next, the instructor can fill his or her lectures with personal anecdotes and experiences that relate to the topic. Hold examinations in suspended animation until the time is suitable for bringing it up. Do not begin an instructional event talking about tests and examinations. Change the environment by going on a field trip or holding lessons outside (weather permitting). Classes that were sometimes held out of doors (this was in the Spring and Fall of the year) was most satisfying and conducive to learning. Pace instruction by making it achievable: not too hard, not too easy, but just right—the Goldilocks zone. Finally, the instructor must understand the interests of his or her learners. Learn about the students in one's class. What are their hobbies? Their goals? Their interests? For example, a college music teacher who was a bit of a character made the most of his students' hobbies and interests. He had a student who was a classical guitarist play some of the music by Sor, Tarrega, and Bach. The class responded enthusiastically. Many of the students had no idea of what classical guitar was; it became a learning experience for them.

EXAMPLES

History

Consider how to select and fit a learning theory to the history example. Based on the title of this unit, The War Between the States: A Southern Perspective, one could recommend a constructivist learning theory. As David (2017) noted "Knowledge is constructed based on personal experiences and hypotheses about the environment. Learners continuously test these hypotheses through social negotiation" (p. 1). The objective of this instructional sequence is both cognitive and affective. We wish to create empathy with a now slandered population and cause. It is extremely important to analyze peoples and events in the context of the times in which they lived.

A secondary choice would be cognitivism. David (2017) observed that "Mental processes such as thinking, memory, knowing, and problem-solving need to be explored. Knowledge can be seen as a schema or symbolic mental constructions. Learning is defined as change in a learner's schemata" (p.35). This unit could be successfully taught without invoking empathy while concentrating on the intellectual aspects of the subject. If so, we might miss an opportunity to present the instruction a manner more congruent with the brain's emotional aspects.

Overall, perhaps the best choice would be to use a constructivist approach. This approach permits students to construct their own knowledge, which will more than likely create strong emotional overtones that will make the learning more meaningful, relevant, timely, and easier to retrieve from memory.

Science

Consider how to select and fit a learning theory to the science example. The topic of this instructional unit is action potentials. This describes the process of generating enough voltage to overcome the maintenance threshold so that the electrical impulse can travel along the neuron to the synaptic gap over which it is transported for transmission along another axon to continue its journey or is terminated in a muscle causing that muscle to contract. The goal for this instructional effort would work under any one of or combination of learning theories: behaviorist, cognitivist, or constructivist. Perhaps the cognitivist theory might prove to be more useful from a cost-benefit perspective.

The action potential could feature animations, video sequences of calcium signaling cells in action, and a WebQuest on YouTube.

Literature

Consider how to select and fit a learning theory to literature. This is somewhat like the history example. Consequently, the constructivist theory holds promise for the topic of literature. One of the genres of folk literature is the ballad. The old ballads tell stories of unrequited love, murder, robbery, and other traumatic events like those we learn about from the news every day. In previous times, such events were captured and shared in the form of songs some of which were composed in medieval times and remain with us today. Many of these old songs are in what is termed modal style, which is a style that is unlike the music we enjoy today. The song, *Scarboro Fair* comes to mind, which is a poignant remembrance of a lost love of long ago in Scarboro. Also, serious events were covered by rather cheerful tunes. For example, try the link to Jimmy Driftwood's rendition of the *Battle of New* Orleans. A similar treatment is afforded the assassination President McKinley as related in the song, *White House Blues*. One of the verses was "McKinley hollered, McKinley squalled, Dr. said McKinley I can't find that ball" played as a rollicking upbeat bluegrass tune. Then, there are folk tales like the *Legend of Sleepy Hollow* and *Rip Van Winkle* that Washington Irving wrote based on a folk story (Glassman, 1985) with humorous overtones. On a more somber note, we have *Young Goodman Brown*, by Nathaniel Hawthorne. This story deals with the Puritan fascination with evil in which all the good people of Brown's home town were in the Devil's clutches. A class could be divided into groups to cover one aspect of these forms of literature, at the end of which they could share their findings with the entire group. It would be particularly nice if some individuals in the class were able to sing and play some of the old ballads.

Archaeology

Consider how to select and fit a learning theory to the archaeology example. This topic would lend itself well to behaviorism or cognitivism owing to the nature of the content, which is the influence of technology in modern archaeology. This could easily lend itself to an unemotional straight forward lecture approach. To give substance to the lecture, an accompanying program such as PowerPoint could contain images and videos of the various applications of technology to find out more about the past of the human family. Also, students could be given the opportunity to use Google Earth to find traces of ancient civilizations. To make the most of this, it would be helpful for specific sites to have already been located by the instructor to which the students could be directed to see for themselves. Video clips of LIDAR and ground-penetrating radar could enhance instruction so that students could see how these devices are used. Also, metal detectors could be shared among the students for a field trip to find artifacts such as Minnie balls from the civil war or treasure hordes in England. Anything to make the presentation come alive would help students to remember the instructional event.

SUMMARY

Despite the great number of learning theories, all of them appear to have varying degrees of validity. Those that seem to subsume most of these elements are the behaviorist, cognitivist, constructivist, and connectivist. One should let the nature of the subject and the nature of his or her learners drive the instruction. The same considerations that drive instruction should be made for the time available for teaching the material, accessibility of resources, and the degree of learner interest in the material. In chapter 5, attention will be focused on instructional design models.

Chapter five treats instructional design theories and models. Seven instructional design models are discussed. The ADDIE approach to designing instruction is covered in some detail. Evaluation of learning is part of the chapter. The role of feedback in the process of learning is covered. Gagné's nine instructional events are also part of the chapter. A table containing the learning theory and associated instructional activities ends the chapter.

REFERENCES

Armstrong, P. (2017). *Bloom's taxonomy.* Vanderbilt University Center for Teaching. Retrieved from https://cft.vanderbilt.edu/guides-sub-pages/blooms-taxo

Bilash, O. (2011, January). Krathwol's affective domain taxonomy. *Best of Bilash*. Retrieved from https://sites.educ.ualberta.ca/staff/olenka.bilash/Best%20of%20Bilash/krathwol.html

Bixler, B. (n.d.). *Action verbs for objectives*. Retrieved from http://www.personal.psu.edu/bxb11/Objectives/ActionVerbsforObjectives.pdf

Brenton, L. (2016). *Top 10 ways to increase your students' interest in a subject*. Retrieved from https://www.emergingedtech.com/2016/04/10-ways-to-increase-students-interest-in-a-subject/

Cherry, K. (2019 July 26). *What Is sociocultural theory?* Retrieved from https://www.verywellmind.com/what-is-sociocultural-theory-2795088

David, L. (2017). *Learning theories in plain English Vol. 1 of 2*. Retrieved from https://www.learning-theories.com/product/learning-theories-in-plain-english-ebook

Four top learning theories in the digital age. (2015). Retrieved from https://www.sanfordbrown.edu/student-life/blog/march-2015/four-top-learning-theories-in-the-age

Glassman, P. (1987). Afterword. In W. Irving, Rip Van Winkle (pp. 87-94). New York, NY: Books of Wonder William Morrow and Company.

Jensen, E. (2008). *Brain-based learning: A new paradigm of teaching* (2nd ed.). Thousand Oaks, CA: Corwin Press.

Laws, G. (2015, September). Psycho-Motor taxonomy: Elizabeth J. Simpson. *Instructional Design*. Retrieved from http://www.geolawsdesign.com/glossary/psycho-motor-taxonomy-elizabeth-j-simpson/

Learning theories. (2019). Retrieved from http://www.about-elearning.com/learning-theories.html

Little, B. (2015). *The top 10 learning theories*. Retrieved from https://www.mindtools.com/blog/corporate/the-top-ten-learning-theories/

Mazer, J. P. (2013). Associations among teacher communication behaviors, student Interest, and engagement: A validity test. *Communication Education*, *62*(1), 86–96. doi:10.1080/03634523.2012.731513

Paul, A. M. (2013). *How to stimulate curiosity*. Retrieved from http://ideas.time.com/2013/04/15/how-to-stimulate-curiosity/

Chapter 5
Instructional Design Models and Theories

ABSTRACT

Instructional design models help instructors to organize, develop, administer, and evaluate learning programs. Seven of the theories that drive these efforts are situated cognition theory, sociocultural learning theory, the ADDIE model, Merrill's principles of instruction, individualized instruction, Bloom's taxonomy of learning objectives, and the SAM model. All these models are highly iterative meaning that changes are frequent and interlocked. This makes the evaluation of learning that occurred highly important. Dr. Robert Mager is credited with being the father of the instructional objective. The effective performance objective consists of three parts: the terminal behavior, the conditions under which the behavior will be performed, and a standard of acceptable performance. Consequently, the complete objective contains the essence of what should be evaluated. A very key element in this learning process is the provision of immediate and detailed feedback. Several good authoring apps exist that can support computers in performing this task.

DOI: 10.4018/978-1-7998-1542-6.ch005

Figure 1.

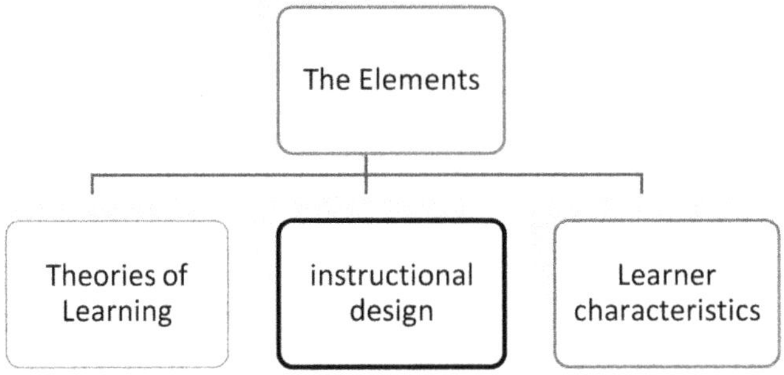

INFORMATION AND COMMUNICATIONS TECHNOLOGY (ICT) CAPABILITY

One must make a distinction between information and communications technology (ICT) capability and instructional technology: ICT subsumes Instructional technology. Nay (2019) divides ICT capability into three areas: investigation, communication, and creation. Though this is ostensibly for lower grades, it is highly likely to transcend grade and age levels. While computer hardware and software experience constant change with old ones becoming obsolete or dropped as new and more sophisticated software are developed, ICT remains relatively constant with its mission of investigation, communication, and creation. It can engage in this mission regardless of specific hardware and software.

ICT plays a key role in education with teaching, learning, and assessment. Among these are the following:

- enhance learning opportunities through access to a range of resources, stimulus materials, and learning tools
- provide increased opportunities for student engagement and motivation
- equip students with the necessary knowledge and skills to use ICT to support 21st-century learning
- support the development of effective student research and evaluation skills
- promote critical and creative thinking skills
- increase teacher and student efficiency
- develop an awareness of the public nature of online activity and related responsibilities

- increase opportunities to work collaboratively, locally, nationally and globally Nay (2019 August 19, para. 3).

ICT can be applied in various forms, some of which are as follows:

- multimedia creation tools, including cameras, microphones, and audio editing programs
- programming tools
- game-based learning and game development opportunities
- online collaboration tools, including blogs and wikis
- web 2.0 and web 3.0 tools
- GPS, geo-tagging, geographic information systems
- simulations
- electronic portfolios
- productivity tools, including word processing, databases, spreadsheets, graphic editing
- interactive manipulatives, such as interactive geometry applications
- contextualised learning experiences, including robotics, 3D modelling, virtual learning environments (including field trips), web quests (Nay, 2019 August 19, para. 5).

Next, one would be wise to explore instructional design models and theories and how to apply them.

INSTRUCTIONAL DESIGN MODELS AND THEORIES

There are a host of instructional design models. An instructional design model, according to Kurt (2015) "… provides guidelines to organize appropriate pedagogical scenarios to achieve instructional goals. Instructional design can be defined as the practice of creating instructional experiences to help facilitate learning most effectively" (para. 1). Kurt (2015) goes on to state that "Instructional design models describe how to conduct the various steps. These steps involve the instructional design process. The models help trainers and educators to guide and plan [the] overall process" (para 1). With respect to the information explosion, instructional design offers a way to make learning more effective and efficient through the application of a systematic and precise process.

INSTRUCTIONAL DESIGN THEORIES

Out of the number of competing theories and models for instructional design, those that are most useful for online course design will be explored. Pappas (September 2, 2017) identified the seven most common instructional design models and theories for online course design.

Situated Cognition Theory

The situated cognition theory was first posed by Brown, Collins, and Duguid (1989) in an article printed in The Educational Researcher. This theory has three primary tenents: 1) knowing and doing cannot be separated; 2) what is learned must be applied in the context in which it was learned; and 3) learning is a social activity that expands knowledge through discussions and group problem-solving tasks (Pappas, September 2, 2017).

Pappas (June 7, 2015) explains its application to online course design

... it is obvious that the Situated Cognition Theory is directly related to the way that eLearning content is presented to the audience. This implies that all type[s] of new information learners are exposed to, should be given within context. In practice, from an instructional designer's point of view, this can be translated to the incorporation of case studies and interactive branching scenarios and simulations of real-life settings in which the particular piece of knowledge would apply. By all means, all eLearning activities should make explicit to the learners the connection of what is actually presented as part of the eLearning content with its practical application in real life. (Pappas, September 2, 2017. p. 4).

Sociocultural Learning Theory

This instructional design learning theory is the product of a Russian psychologist named Leo Vygotsky. Though written in 1934, the works of Vygotsky did not reach the Western world until 1978 owing to its suppression by Stalin. Pappas (November 26, 2014) noted that,

The Sociocultural Learning Theory is based upon the idea that a learner's environment plays a pivotal role in his/her learning development. According to Vygotsky the learning process actually involves three key themes: culture, language, and the "zone of proximal development (The Quintessential of the Sociocultural Learning Theory, para. 2).

Vygotsky noted that cultures are the result of humans using tools and symbols. Language, as noted by the sociocultural learning theory, is a direct result of the tools and symbols that develop from culture. The zone of proximal development describes the gap that lies between possible development and actual development.

Pappas goes on to describe the application of the sociocultural learning theory as taking

... into account how learners are impacted by their peers, and how social scenarios impact their ability to acquire information. As such, instructors who apply the Sociocultural Learning Theory in their instructional design can also become aware of how learners may directly impact one another, as well as how cultural "norms" can influence a learner's learning behavior. They can then create an eLearning course plan that integrates the principles of Sociocultural Learning, in order to enhance the effectiveness of the curriculum (The Quintessential of the Sociocultural Learning Theory. para. 7).

The ADDIE Model

This is likely the most recognizable model for most instructional designers. The acronym, ADDIE, stands for Analyze, Design, Develop, Implement, and Evaluate. This model was developed in 1975 at Florida State University by the U. S. Army to be used to train members of the military both efficiently and effectively for various military ratings, many of them quite complex (Pappas, September 2, 2017). Pappas (September 2, 2017) noted that "ADDIE tackles eLearning development rather than learning behaviors. It allows Instructional Designers to delve into the needs, learning objectives, and desired outcomes so as to create more personalized eLearning resources" (The ADDIE Model, para. 5).

Merrill's Principles of Instruction

Merrill's theory focuses on four core phases of learning: "demonstration, activation of previous knowledge, application, integration into real-world challenges" (Pappas, September 2, 2017, para. 5). This theory also incorporates scaffolding through which learners move from simpler to more complex ideas and concepts as the instruction continues (Pappas, September 2, 2017, Merrill's principles of instruction, para. 5).

Individualized Instruction

The individualized instruction theory revolves around individuals and how they learn. This means that students who quickly catch on to the content presented in the lesson can progress rapidly, while those students who fail to immediately catch on can take the time to go over and review the material as much as needed until they too can move forward. According to Pappas (September 2, 2017) the individualized instruction theory rests upon four principles:

1. Learners should be able to complete the work autonomously. As a result, they can focus on their own strengths and areas for improvement.
2. Each lesson should be followed by an assessment to gauge learner progress.
3. Written learning materials are preferred over presentations.
4. Facilitators support learners and add a level of social interactivity to the experience (para. 6).

The individualized instruction method is designed to match the educational needs and skills of individual learners. Matching these needs and skills involves varying the pace with which the instruction is delivered, offering different methods for delivering the content (differentiated instruction), and how the materials are distributed. Students receive detailed and generally effective media or textbooks with a minimum of lecture and presentation. Learners receive encouragement to review, research, and learn the material at their own pace.

Bloom's Taxonomy of Learning Objectives

Bloom and his team created this theory in the 1950s (Pappas, 2013). It consists of three learning domains: cognitive, affective, and psychomotor. While Bloom focused on the cognitive domain, others have modified it and created taxonomies for the psychomotor and affective domains. Each domain contains a hierarchy of levels of performance from the lowest to the highest. These domains provide various action verbs that can be incorporated into performance objectives.

The SAM Model

SAM stands for the successive approximation model. The essential characteristic of this model is that it permits instructional designers to make changes through small steps and numerous iterations. Pappas (2017). Another model is very similar to it:

The Spiral Model centers on risks. More specifically, how to minimize risks so that your eLearning course achieves the desired results. The client is involved in every step of the way to improve the eLearning course design and remedy unforeseen issues. Barry Boehm first introduced the Spiral Model back in 1988 [1], which combines iterative and sequential linear approaches. It was originally intended for software development and testing. However, it has since become popular in Instructional Design. The Spiral Model consists of four main stages: planning, risk analysis, engineering or content creation, and evaluation. (How To Apply The Spiral Model Of Iterative Design In eLearning, para. 1).

The spiral model is typically applied through eight steps:

1. Identify the needs and create a budget for your eLearning project
2. Set A Realistic Design and Development Schedule
3. Create Communication Guidelines
4. Determine the Risks Involved and Create A Plan B
5. Develop A Phased Prototype
6. Gather Client's Feedback at Each Stage
7. Re-Assess the Risks Periodically
8. Use Client's Input to Continually Improve Your eLearning Course Design (Pappas, May 12, 2013, How to Apply The Spiral Model Of Iterative Design In eLearning).

Communities of Inquiry (CoI): Refers to a three-element model of overlapping circles consisting of social presence, cognitive presence, and teaching presence. See Figure 2. One might wonder what the phrase, Cognitive Presence means. Garrison (Cited in Broda, 2018) defines Cognitive Presence as "…a process of inquiry that includes thinking, listening and expressing thoughts in the process of critical discourse" (para. 2). Social presence is defined as the "dialogically inquisitive, active and reflective, articulate, cognitively adept, cooperative, sensitive to context, and explorative" (Cited

Figure 2. Community of inquiry

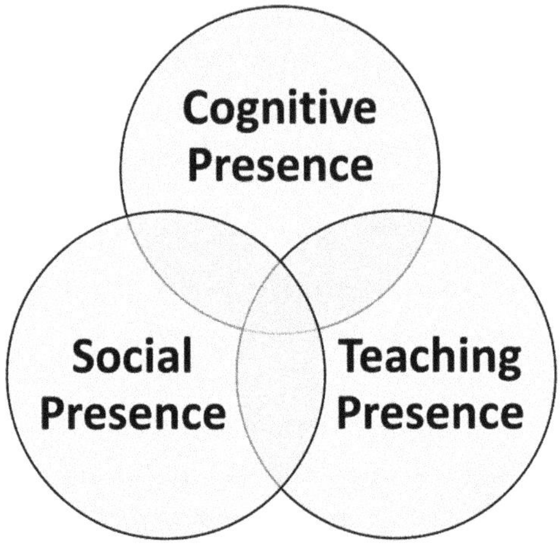

in Broda, 2018). The third element of the triad, teaching presence, is defined as the "the design, facilitation, and direction of [student] cognitive and social processes for the purpose of realizing personally meaningful and educationally worthwhile learning outcomes" (Pearson, 2018).

Social Presence

- Engagement with participants
- Risk-free expression
- Encouraging collaboration

Teaching Presence

- Setting the curriculum
- Sharing personal meaning
- Focusing discussion (Adapted from Broda (2018 October 2))

Where the Cognitive Presence and the Social Presence overlap, one finds Supporting Discourse. The overlap of Social Presence and Teaching presence receives the label, Setting Climate. The overlap between Teaching Presence and Cognitive presence is labeled as Selecting Content. The center where all circles overlap is titled the Educational Experience. This model is particularly good for use in online courses.

Action Research

Action research is a discipline in which the actor is engaged in a close examination of a topic of inquiry. The process consists of seven steps:

1. Selecting a focus
2. Clarifying theories
3. Identifying research questions
4. Collecting data
5. Analyzing data
6. Reporting results
7. Taking informed action (Sagor, 2019, para. 2).

The purposes of action research reflect the flexibility of its application to the individual teacher, or a collaboration of colleagues, or even the entire faculty of a school or educational organization (Sagor, 2019). Consequently, three purposes are "building the reflective practitioner, making progress on schoolwide priorities, and building professional cultures" (Sagor, 2019, para, 10). Action research is imminently practical and is assuming greater practical importance as time passes.

GAGNÉ'S NINE INSTRUCTIONAL EVENTS

These instructional events are based upon the conditions of learning that he identified. These five conditions of learning are verbal information, intellectual skills, cognitive strategies, motor skills, and attitudes. Each type of learning requires different external and internal conditions (Culatta, 2019). These conditions lead to the nine events of instruction that can be applied to virtually any pedagogical style either totally or selected elements of it. Four principles were derived from the conditions of learning:

1. Different instruction is required for different learning outcomes.
2. Events of learning operate on the learner in ways that constitute the conditions of learning.
3. The specific operations that constitute instructional events are different for each different type of learning outcome.
4. Learning hierarchies define what intellectual skills are to be learned and a sequence of instruction (Culatta, 2019. Para. 6).

It is from these conditions of learning that Gagné derived the nine instructional events. Culatta (2019), observed that "Gagne´ stated that these nine events could be applied to any type of teaching activity and learning, even if their use and order are different" (p. 770). These nine events are as follows:

1. Gaining attention
2. Informing learners of the objective
3. Stimulating recall of prior learning
4. Presenting the stimulus
5. Providing "learning guidance"
6. Eliciting performance
7. Providing feedback
8. Assessing performance
9. Enhancing retention and transfer (Gagné, 1985. pp. 246-254).

Culatta (2014) noted that "… the original form of Gagne´'s model has a great level of flexibility and is appropriate for four out of five components of the instructional environment (instructor/teacher, learner, subject matter and method) (p. 770). It is very popular among instructional designers and can be applied to the teaching element of virtually all instructional design models and theories.

SELECTING AND APPLYING INSTRUCTIONAL DESIGN MODELS

While several models may be used with equal utility, it is helpful to select one overriding theory or model to guide the design of a project. More than one theory may be used with equal effectiveness. For example, the ADDIE model can easily incorporate Bloom's taxonomy for the cognitive domain, or Krathwohl's affective domain, or Simpson's psychomotor domain, or a combination of these. Selection should be governed by two primary questions: What will be taught? To whom is the instruction directed?

The subject matter of what is to be taught is probably the most complicated question. First one must create behavioral objectives that are precise and measurable. This can be primarily cognitive with a flavoring of affective elements. For example, let us consider the history of the American Civil War. This can contain such cognitive elements as the causes of the war. Affective elements could include how the war impacted the Northern and Southern women of the time; those whose husbands and sweethearts were called to fight the battles, while they were left at home to face the issues of everyday life. Then, we could examine the attitudes of the slaves and the impact of slavery on their existence. Even the psychomotor domain could be invoked by participating in a reenactment of one of the battles of the war. Objectives for this could be summarized as in table 1.

One can see how objectives of the various domains for a variety of subjects could be created and easily evaluated. The objective should contain enough information to guide the development of an evaluation element. For example, in the cognitive objective, one can easily request an analysis of three causes of the war. The same applies to the objective of the affective domain by putting the learner in the place of an individual who lived during those tumultuous times. The psychomotor objective can be evaluated by simply having each student individually and collectively perform the rebel yell.

In the foregoing example, one can readily see how the ADDIE model, Bloom's Taxonomy of Learning Objectives, the SAM model, Individualized Instruction, Merrill's Principles of Instruction, Situated Cognition Theory, and Sociocultural Learning Theory could all be used to design instructional courses and units. A selection from these that could be used might be determined by the characteristics of the learners and the nature of the content, the amount of time available for instruction, and resources to be applied to instruction.

Iterative in Nature Illustrated by the ADDIE Model

The design of instructional material and methods is highly iterative in which each element influences all other elements in response to changes that must inevitably take place. For example, consider an instructional unit on action

Table 1. An example of objectives in three domains

Domain	Objective Example
The cognitive domain at the analysis level.	Given the content in the textbook, analyze three causes of the War Between the States
The affective domain at the responding level.	Given the findings of your research on the causes of the War Between the States by discussing the roles of economics, politics, and slavery in the causes of the war.
The psychomotor domain at the practicing level.	Given the material presented on the Youtube site, The Rebel Yell Lives: Part I - Rediscovering History, perform the rebel yell used by charging Confederate forces.

potentials on the cellular level in human physiology. Using the ADDIE model in which the first A represents analysis, we must first consider the learners. What is their education level? University students? Medical students? A different approach would be required for each of these populations. Furthermore, we must analyze the content in the context of creating learning objectives, of resources, time available for instruction, and the nature of the content. Having completed this step, we begin to design the instructional sequence. How this is designed depends upon the results of our analyses.

This leads to the first D in the ADDIE model: design the instructional approach. One most likely would begin by selecting a learning theory that is suitable for achieving the objectives of instruction. One can create these objectives through the use of the various taxonomies for the cognitive, psychomotor, and affective domains. Ideally, these objectives should consist of three parts: Performance (that which is to be performed), conditions (the conditions under which the performance takes place), and criteria (the level of performance that is deemed acceptable). One can see how the task is becoming more and more complicated.

Next is a move to the second D in the ADDIE model: develop. The next step after designing the instructional sequence is to develop the unit and the instructional material to be used in it. This depends upon available resources. For example, are computers readily available, does everyone have access to the Internet? Are we entirely dependent on less sophisticated resources? The answers to these questions will determine how one starts the design phase.

The I in the ADDIE model represents the implementation of the instructional event. Here, it is wise, to begin with a Beta test (i.e. formative evaluation). This allows the designers to try the new system to identify any problems that are inherent in the first application of any new material. Once the first or first of several offerings of the material have been made, the results analyzed and fixes made, wholesale implementation of the new instruction is started. Even so, other issues will invariably arise that require revisions or workarounds.

The E in the ADDIE model represents evaluation. There are two forms of evaluation: formative and summative; there are two objects of evaluation: the instructional program and learner achievement. Formative evaluation applies to both objects of evaluation, as does summative evaluation. Formative evaluation is that which takes place while the instructional program is being created and when students undertake the instruction as it is taking place. The summative evaluation takes place after everything is up and running. Even though the evaluation takes place at the end of a cycle, it still provides valuable information upon which to revise the program or for students to see where they need additional instruction.

Evaluation of Learning

The means of evaluating an objective should be contained within the objective. Robert F. Mager (1962), often considered the father of the instructional objective, maintains that each objective should consist of three elements: the terminal behavior, the conditions under which the behavior will be performed, and the criterion of acceptable performance. Take an example from his book (Mager, 1962): "Given one or more instructional objectives, you will select those given in performance terms" (p. 1). This objective is complete to the extent that one can easily assess student performance on this subject. Further, in constructing instructional objectives, it is helpful to turn to the taxonomy of educational objectives compiled by Dr. Bloom for the cognitive domain, Dr. Krathwohl's affective domain, or Dr. Simpson's psychomotor domain. When properly written, student learning can be easily tested.

Evaluation of learning can be formative or summative. Formative evaluation is that which occurs during the presentation of instruction. For example, the teacher or facilitator can observe their students to see whether they understand the material. Puzzled expressions, visible confusion, and blank looks can alert the teacher that the material was not understood. This casual formative evaluation permits the teacher to state the material in a different form. Another kind of formative evaluation is a beta test. The beta test is a version of a program that the designers try out to discover problems and other issues that need to be corrected before releasing the material or program. Formative evaluation, then, is conducted as the material is taught,

The summative evaluation takes place once the instruction has been completed. It is designed to determine the degree to which the material has been learned. While it is too late to modify for the group of learners on which it was tested, the results of summative evaluation can be used to improve future versions of the material or the course. One form of summative evaluation is the standardized achievement tests that students take during their academic careers. The SAT and the College Entrance Examination Board (CEEB) are summative evaluations.

Feedback

Timely and accurate feedback is of great value in learning. Feedback must also be specific. Take a simple example: a cook touches a hot pan; the feedback is immediate—the cook quickly withdraws the hand from the hot pan. Learning feedback should also be virtually immediate. If the delay is too long, the link between the action and the reaction may be slowed to the point of insignificance. It can be so delayed that the errant behavior must be unlearned and replaced with the appropriate response, which is likely more difficult than learning the correct way in the first place. This is certainly true in music instrument performance.

Computing technology has grown so sophisticated that immediate feedback can be designed into instructional programs. Schroeder (2018) of eLearning Industry lists 12 authoring programs and provides a link (https://elearningindustry.com/directory/software-categories/elearning-authoring-tools) from his post to the eLearning Industry site that lists 95 authoring programs. Also, various learning management systems (LMS) have built-in authoring programs. Many of these programs have templates to help you get a head start on projects.

For example, such authoring programs make it possible to apply Gagne's (1985) nine instructional events as depicted in table 2.

The nine steps are easily divided into three sections: preparation, instruction, and practice, assessment and transfer. Preparation includes the first three sections. Instruction and practice include four, five, six, and seven instructional events. Assessment and transfer include the final two sections, which are eight and nine for the results.

EXAMPLES

History, Science, Literature, and Archaeology

These units could be delivered in a way that is congruent with several learning theories and instructional design models. Four of them come to mind: behaviorist, constructivist, cognitivist, and connectivist. See table 3 to see how these might work.

Table 2. Gagné's nine instructional events

Instructional Event	Authoring Program Ability	Purpose
1. Gain attention	The authoring program could present a brief visual sequence germane to the lesson	To provide a for context the lesson.
2. Share objective	The objective of the lesson could be announced as a voice-over of the text of the objective.	Make the student aware of what is expected.
3. Stimulate recall of prior learning	A screen could present something that the student already knows or with which he or she is familiar.	To remind the student of having learned the three chords.
4. Present stimulus	Screens present the material that the student is expected to learn.	The stimulus is provided via the example.
5. Provide learner guidance	A voice-over could lead the student through several examples of what is to be learned.	Provide verbal instructions and demonstrations.
6. Elicit performance	A branching sequence could be used in which the student could be asked to select appropriate responses.	To demonstrate success in learning the piece.
7. Give feedback	Immediate feedback is possible given a branch that reflects each choice the student makes.	This feedback enhances learning.
8. Assess performance	Administer a computer-based test that provides an immediate response to either each choice or at the end of the test.	It helps the student to perform the piece correctly.
9. Enhance retention and Recall	Provide other examples that illustrate the topic of the lesson.	To apply the material learned to a real-life situation.

Connelly & Miller (2018)

SUMMARY

Instructional design theories and the models derived from them perform a valuable service in creating instructional sequences and materials. The theory or model selected should be suitable for the objectives and content of the proposed instructional event. These models and theories are highly iterative, meaning that they are all interlocked and a change in one part often creates changes in other parts. The ADDIE model provides a good illustration of how instructional sequences or units are created. Evaluating learning heavily depends on accurate and well-written learning objectives. Timely and specific feedback is crucial to making learning more efficient and effective. For example, Gagne's nine instructional events demonstrate the entire instructional event, including evaluation.

Chapter 6 concerns learner characteristics. Four topics are dealt with: student characteristics, technical characteristics, administrative characteristics,

Table 3. Applying instructional methods in accordance with four learning theories

Theory	Application
Behaviorist	Present the material as programmed instruction in which small bits of information is imparted and followed immediately with interaction points.
Constructivist	The class is divided into groups each of which will examine one of the objectives, arrive as a team at a conclusion, and present their findings to the entire class.
Cognitivist	The class will participate as a group in the instructional process with an emphasis on making internal mental connections with the subject content.
Connectivist	The class will work either individually or in small teams to conduct WebQuests and to contact others in the field of study to discover what they have concluded and how they arrived at that conclusion.

and issues regarding motivation. Examples of academic subject matter are provided.

REFERENCES

Connelly, J. O., & Miller, P. (2018). Improving learning outcomes for higher education through smart technology. *International Journal of Conceptual Structures and Smart Applications*, *6*(1), 1–17. doi:10.4018/IJCSSA.2018010101

Culatta, R. (2019). *Conditions of learning (Robert Gagne).* Retrieved from https://www.instructionaldesign.org/theories/conditions-learning/

Gagné, R. M. (1985). *The conditions of learning and theory of instruction* (4th ed.). New York, NY: Holt, Rinehart, and Winston.

Kurt, S. (2015). *Instructional design models and theories.* Retrieved from https://educationaltechnology.net/instructional-design-models-and-theories/

Mager, R. F. (1962). *Preparing instructional objectives.* Palo Alto, CA: Fearon.

Nay, A. (2019 August 19). *K-6 learning resources.* Retrieved from https://audreynay.weebly.com/#

Pappas, C. (2014, November 26). *Instructional design models and theories: The sociocultural learning theory.* Retrieved from https://elearningindustry.com/sociocultural-learning-theory

Pappas, C. (2015, June). *Instructional design models and theories: The situated cognition theory and the cognitive apprenticeship model.* Retrieved from https://elearningindustry.com/situated-cognition-theory-and-cognitive-apprenticeship-model

Pappas, C. (2017, September 2). *Elearning course design: 7 instructional design theories & models to consider.* Retrieved from https://elearning.adobe.com/2017/11/elearning-course-design-7-instructional-design-theories-models-consider/

Schroeder, P. (2018, January 22). *Choosing an instructional design software 101.* Retrieved from https://elearningindustry.com/instructional-design-software-101-choose-right

Chapter 6
Learner Characteristics for Online Learning

ABSTRACT

Learner characteristics are vital to student success so that teachers can reach them and stimulate their curiosity such that they will wish to learn and find it interesting. One characteristic unique to the online venue is students feeling isolated. Other distinguishing elements include the type of course, whether students pay for their courses, demographics, self-efficacy, motivation, and control over the learning process. Technical characteristics also affect online learning. These characteristics include user-friendly technology, convenience, sophisticated technology, previous experience with eLearning, and access to mobile technology. Administrative characteristics are also important and include nine constituent elements. These include affective learning engagement and the success of community colleges. Then one must consider recognition of essential learner traits, learning styles, motivational factors, the situation theory of publics, and the role of self-efficacy. Next, administration should promote self-regulatory learning skills and improved course access. Finally, motivation characteristics must also be considered. All of these elements influence student success in online learning.

DOI: 10.4018/978-1-7998-1542-6.ch006

LEARNER CHARACTERISTICS FOR ONLINE LEARNING

A multitude of learner characteristics suggested success in online learning. Among these was the need to feel part of the class. The online setting is one of social isolation owing to the nature of the setting. Students who feel isolated are not likely to do well online (Seiver & Troja, 2014; Aversa & MacCall, 2013; Waladis, Hachy, & Conway, 2013). For example, Seiver and Troja (2014) pointed out that the likelihood of success depended upon how connected participants felt to their classmates and their instructor. They supported this observation through references to various studies. In their estimation, the best academic performance was the result of instructors who facilitated social interaction; the greatest satisfaction was the result of collaboration with classmates. "The greatest predictor of student satisfaction were [sic] instructor feedback, clear directions from the instructor, and clear expectations of course work" (Seiver & Troja, 2014, p. 91). See Table 1 for a listing of learner characteristics.

Isolation among online learners creates a problem that can interfere with learning. Aversa and MacCall (2013) based their efforts on ways to combat the negative effects of isolation among online students. Among these efforts were activities such as providing opportunities for group work, communication (in and outside of class activities), and social opportunities. Additional efforts included making programs and other university activities available to online students. Further, guest speakers, faculty job candidate presentations, and workshops were routinely provided for online students. Faculty and staff availability at informal and formal social gatherings, at professional conferences, and meetings around the country were also provided. Even with all these opportunities, academic rigor was kept equivalent to that of face to

Figure 1.

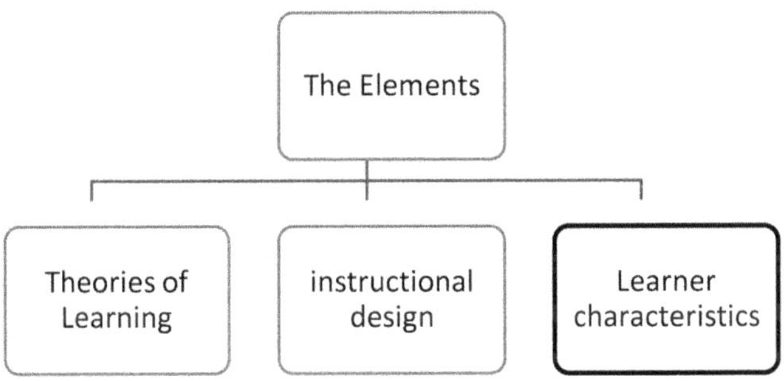

Table 1. Learner characteristics affecting student success in online learning

Characteristic	Purpose
Connectedness to classmates and instructor	To reduce the isolation that is inherent in online venues through group work, social opportunities, guest speakers, and so forth.
Type of course	In STEM courses for non-majors, target and provide support to persist and to succeed in them.
Pay for courses	People tend to value that for which they pay and hold in little esteem that for which they do not pay.
Successful completion of previous online courses.	If a student has successfully completed an online course, it tends to promote completion of another online course.
Demographics: female, older, married, part-time students	These demographics tend to describe those who enroll in online courses.
Self-efficacy	Students having strong self-efficacy and self-regulation tend to do well in online courses.
Student Motivation	Students are motivated to learn by six factors: external motivators, curiosity, self-efficacy, attitude, need, and competence (Rovai et al. 2007). Further, online students appear to be more strongly motivated than traditional classroom students.
Direct and control the learning process particularly time and resources.	Online university students seem to direct and control their learning processes, time, and resources.

face classes. These efforts seem to have borne positive as evidenced by high retention among these online students.

Wladis, Hachy, and Conway (2013) explored the efficacy of online student success for those who enrolled in science, technology, engineering, and mathematics (STEM) courses. As might be expected, there were significant differences depending upon the kind of STEM courses that were taken by online students. They concluded that "… students enrolled in online STEM courses, particularly when they are introductory courses or taken by a large proportion of students as electives or distributional requirements for non-STEM majors, may need targeted support in order to persist and succeed" (p. 80). For example, instructors could provide training programs with links to optimize the student's strategies. Also, student support services could be integrated into the online learning context to connect them with resources for learning. Further, targeted support could include online tutorials with assessments of their potential for success.

Other elements influenced student success in online learning. Philip and Lee (2011) found two elements that affected student success in online learning: participants who paid for their courses as opposed to those who did not; participants who posted a photograph of themselves in their personal profiles. Philip and Lee (2011) discovered that students who paid for their courses were more likely to pass (37.8%) their courses than those who paid no tuition (16%), while those whose tuition was waived scored lowest of all (12.5%). These characteristics would suggest that those who paid were more likely to place greater value on that for which they paid. In this same study, those who had successfully passed a previous online course were likely to complete additional online courses at 41.5% as opposed to 19.9% of those who had not previously taken such a course. This seems to suggest that those who are engaged in the course were more likely to complete it successfully. Interestingly, those who posted a photograph of themselves in their personal profile passed at 42.1% as opposed to 22.4% who had not uploaded a photograph of themselves.

Having taken previous online courses seemed to have made a difference in student success in current courses. One might reasonably think that previous experience with online courses and relative facility with such technology would produce highly effective studying by online students; however, that is not necessarily the case. Liaw (as cited in Bouhnik and Golan, 2012) noted "...that internet experience doesn't necessarily affect the E-learning quality. He claims that what is most important is the level of functionality and interaction the website has with the students" (p. 20). Further, Bouhnik and Golan (2012) found, concerning previous experience with online courses, the sole significant outcome concerning prior study in earlier E-courses and improved thinking dispositions was "...among students who had no prior E-course experience" (p. 30).

Previous experience with online learning seemed to make a difference in the degree of satisfaction a learner feels about a course. Cortés and Barberá (2013) examined time patterns and perceptions of online learning success. They discovered that students who spent more than 12 hours per day online experienced greater knowledge transfer than those who spent three to five hours per day online. Furthermore, those spending more time online during the day promoted greater knowledge transfer, especially during the morning hours. The concluding observation about learner satisfaction was that those with greater experience with the internet have more confidence using the learning platform and completing course tasks. On the other hand, Hachey, Wladis, and Conway (2012) concluded from their study that online course experience plays a major role in future online success. Students not having completed previous online courses have very low retention and success.

Cao and Sakchutchawan (2011) examined three research questions concerning MBA students. Concerning demographics "Female, older, married and part-time adult MBA students are more likely to choose online courses"

(p. 7). Student success as measured through grades show no significant difference between face to face and online learners. Concerning course satisfaction, online students tended to be less satisfied with their learning experience than students who met in face to face classes. Nevertheless, the authors concluded, "…that the doubts and negative perceptions of employers and even faculty on the quality and overall value of online MBA education have no strong basis" (p.10).

Self-efficacy plays a role in student success. Concerning the use of mobile technology for learning, the Unified Theory of Acceptance and Use of Technology (UTAUT) model provided insight regarding four elements and their impact on acceptance and learning: performance expectancy, effort expectancy, social influence, and facilitating conditions (Irby & Strong, 2015). They noted that "Mobile learning may be perceived as a more attractive task by highly self-efficacious students, but not those with low self-efficacy. Students with low self-efficacy may be wary of confronting even a familiar technology like mobile technology" (Irby & Strong 2015, p. 14). Though this study focused on mobile technology, one could likely conclude that it would also apply to the standard computer configuration of online learning.

Student motivation played a significant role in successful online learning. Rovai, Ponton, Wighting, and Baker (2007) concluded that online students demonstrate stronger motivation than on-campus face to face students on three intrinsic motivation scales: to know, to accomplish, and to experience stimulation. They noted no difference on three scales that measured external motivation and no motivation. The e-learning students reported learning to be more gratifying and they had greater satisfaction from the methods, activities, and practices of learning (Rovai et al., 2007). For example, e-learners could study content and apply their knowledge to collaborative online questions and reports. In addition, lessons were adaptable for easy viewing on computers, mobile devices, smartphones, and tablets (Centers for Disease Control and Prevention, 2013). According to Rovai et al., (2007), students who complete online courses are intrinsically motivated to make this achievement.

Learning strategies and learning satisfaction create a positive relationship for strengthening online learning. Choi (2016) examined the relationship between graduate students' learning strategies and learning satisfaction. Choi determined that learning in an online environment is largely dependent upon the student's ability to direct and control the learning process, particularly time and resources. The students in online programs, as an example, are encouraged to study with a certain level of inquiry, examination, and analysis. Successful learners participate and share their knowledge in many structured learning activities. The learners participate in reflective questions, dialogue among classmates, substantive responses, weekly reflections, as well as individual forums for group assignments. The conclusion was that successful online learning must include each learner's metacognition and engagement in peer learning.

TECHNICAL CHARACTERISTICS

The technical aspects of online learning have serious ramifications for students enrolled in these courses. It is important to eliminate as many barriers as possible that stand between the learner and the course material. Consequently, the technology should be easy to use and reliable. Stark, Lassiter, and Kuemper (2013) had as the primary goal of their examination to determine the kinds of support needed to help lower-level and upper-level learners to succeed in online learning. Their research suggests that access to technology was more helpful for lower-level learners, while motivation and self-discipline were more helpful for upper-level learners, while neither access to technology nor experience with technology affected student performance. Therefore, administrators of online programs should select reliable and easy to use course management systems. Further, course designers and facilitators should recognize barriers and seek to use available resources to overcome these barriers. See Table 2 for a listing of technical characteristics.

Various studies (as cited in Salyers, Carter, Carter, Myers, & Barrett, 2014) noted that university students and returning adult learners turn to e-learning for two reasons: convenience and technological sophistication. Further, they note that for effectiveness the e-learning environments should "…1) address the

Table 2. Technical characteristics affecting student success in online learning

Characteristics	Purpose
Easy to use technology	Put the focus on the content of the learning rather than on the technology.
Convenience	The technology must be intuitive so that little if any, mental effort is put on using the technology.
Technological sophistication	The technology must match the actions expected of students and teachers who are using it.
Previous experience with eLearning	This previous experience will reduce or eliminate becoming familiar with the way the system works.
Mobile technology access	This makes it possible for students to learn at any time and in any place.

needs of e-learners, 2) apply effective pedagogical strategies, 3) incorporate state of the art instructional design principles, 4) support multiple technologies, and 5) provide for flexible and interactive learning opportunities" (para. 12). They strongly noted that such technical elements as ease of navigation, course design, and previous e-learning experience were important predictive variables that contributed to the success of e-learning students. Further, it suggested that teaching and learning needed to be combined with the technological components of instructional delivery. Two additional important components were immediacy and social presence. Previous experience with e-learning also proved to be a strong predictor of future success in online learning.

Mobile telecommunications access has developed rapidly over the years. Arndt & Guercio, (2014) explored the role of ubiquitous e-learning in the context of online e-learning. Ubiquity is defined as snatching the odd time or times during the day to engage in e-learning via various e-learning telecommunications devices. These devices include iPhones and other similar mobile devices. They concluded that students who have mobile devices use them throughout the day when they can catch a few minutes to engage in their course work. This action allows learners to make use of virtually every idle moment to engage with the learning available through their online programs of study.

ADMINISTRATIVE CHARACTERISTICS

Administrative characteristics exert a profound influence on the success of students in the online classroom. Kamali (2014) suggested that whether e-learning will replace the learning that takes place in a traditional classroom remains questionable; however, other forces will likely exert influences that make e-learning an irreversible trend. The foundation of learning, in their opinion, resides in affective learning engagement (ALE) in either or both face to face and online learning. According to the Centers for Disease Control and Prevention (2013), learners must focus on the knowledge and skills to be learned with objectives that are measurable and approaches that support the learning. Students can develop methods for successfully engaging in their courses and building an effective team for group assignments. Learning teams are one way that students discover methods that are used to communicate effectively, develop a contract, and benefit by sharing their skills among group members. See Table 3 for a listing of administrative characteristics that affect student success in online learning.

Table 3. Administrative characteristics affecting student success in online learning

Characteristic(s)	Purpose
Affective learning engagement	Administration should initiate and support learning engagement by the student.
Address and recognize essential learner characteristics	Make a successful effort to know the characteristics of your students.
Learning styles	Pay reasonable attention to the learning styles of the various students.
Motivational elements	Consider and invoke motivational factors in online learning environments.
Consider the role of self-efficacy	Consider and use the role of self-efficacy in online classes because online study depends heavily on this variable.
Promote self-regulatory learning skills	Promote self-regulatory learning skills because students who find themselves in the relatively isolated milieu of online courses must become responsible for their own learning.

The role of the community college in online learning should not be underrated. Hachey, Conway, and Wladis (2013) presented the view of these institutions. The community college seems to serve a demographic that is less prepared for the academic requirements of higher education, which produces a high dropout rate for these students. Nevertheless, the online venue appears to be the more desirable option for further education. This provides the administration with a need to examine their databases to find ways to accommodate this group of learners. Hachey, Conway, and Wladis (2013) noted that “Policies and resource allocations supported by such research will improve the chances of reaching the ultimate goal-- optimizing student success” (para. 24).

The administration should recognize and address essential learner characteristics. Floyd, Harrington, and Santiago (as cited in Kianmehr & Kamali, 2013) perceived that course value and student engagement were the primary supports for student interest. Also, Diaz and Entonado (cited in Kianmehr & Kamali, 2013) contended that even though the facilitator’s role in delivering course content is vital to student learning. Likewise, it also depends upon the effort of the student’s affective learning engagement (ALE) and their active participation in learning scenarios. Kianmehr and Kamali (2013) concluded that it is important to recognize and address the essential characteristic of learners. This element may mitigate against a high rate of course failure, dropping courses, or incomplete grades.

One would likely think that addressing various learning styles would be a logical approach to take; however, this is not necessarily the case. Gappi (2013) sought to determine if there was a relationship between student learning styles and academic success and satisfaction in online courses. This study concluded that there were no significant differences between these variables. The logical assumption would be that students who exhibit various learning styles (i.e. visual, auditory, kinesthetic) can succeed in online courses. It is likely that some degree of adaptation would occur to accommodate the various learning styles (e.g. such as providing transcripts for visual material and providing illustrative visual material for text material). However, these adaptations or accommodations are likely to be successful with little difficulty.

Administrators should realize that they can make use of various motivational elements to encourage students. Smith (2010) examined the role of motivational factors in successful e-learning. The study suggested that motivation does not necessarily follow good quality instruction. Three theories of increasing motivation were explored: Keller's ARC model (attention, relevance, confidence, and satisfaction), Wlodkowski's time continuum model of motivation, and the social cognitive learning theory. Smith (2010) noted that "Ultimately, instructors and machine-based instruction cannot control learner motivation, but on the other hand, they cannot avoid influencing the motivation of learners, either positively or negatively" (p. 7). Wendt and Wendt (2012) determined, concerning motivation to succeed in online courses, that many factors affect motivation, such as prompt feedback and prompt responses to questions, building a community of learners, and the use of formal and informal support systems that help students.

Kruger-Ross and Waters (2013) approached the issue through the Situation Theory of Publics. To define this theory: "The situational theory of publics consists of three independent variables (problem recognition, constraint recognition and level of involvement) and two dependent variables (information seeking and information processing)" (as cited in Kruger-Ross & Waters, 2013, p. 178). The study demonstrated that the Situation Theory of Publics revealed "how students' awareness of the course concepts, how they approached recognized constraints and sought to overcome them, and how they were involved in the course, but also were very accurate in predicting test scores" (p. 181).

Administrators can influence the quality of the online experience for students. Alqurashi (2016) conducted a literature review to discover the findings concerning any relationship that might exist between self-efficacy and online learning environments. This review produced a variety of texts that primarily examined the role of technology and computing as a source of self-efficacy. Alqurashi examined the role of four factors and their relationship to self-efficacy: academic, computer, prior online learning, and student satisfaction. A positive significant relationship was found among computer self-efficacy, prior experience, and student satisfaction. Alqurashi (2016) concluded that more research is needed to determine the role of self-efficacy. Computers, the Internet, and information finding skills are important as are learning, interaction, and collaboration skills.

One would likely wonder whether previous high school experience with online learning would make a significant difference in their college work. Kirby, Barbour, and Sharpe (2015) discovered, essentially, that self-regulatory learning behaviors in online courses were equally apparent in students who had never had an online course compared to those who had. There are many methods for promoting self-regulated learning skills for achievement. The e-learners should have basic computer and technical skills to function effectively online. In addition, learners need a degree of information literacy to maximize their success for their program of study. This means that e-learners need to grasp information that is conveyed with an ability to research the topic, search for materials, and evaluate the subject matter (Clark & Fishleigh, 2012).

Previous success in online courses has shown positive outcomes in community college. Xu and Jaggars (2013) concluded that students who do well in online courses tend to be better prepared and more motivated to succeed in such courses. Online courses tended to improve course access and flexibility. For example, online classes can fit around work and family responsibilities. Online education provides students with the opportunity to study in rural areas without long-distance commutes. Online education has made it possible for anyone to go back to school with a schedule that meets their needs. From the student perspective, these conveniences offered by online courses are both valuable to adult learners and can be a benefit to workforce development.

MOTIVATION CHARACTERISTICS

Motivation plays an important role in the successful completion of online courses. Motivation has traditionally been classed into two categories: extrinsic motivation and intrinsic motivation. The role of student motivation in online course success remains somewhat elusive. Nevertheless, the role of motivation must be considered in any online course offerings. Such motivation may include making it easy for students to interact and collaborate on assignments (Bettinger, Liu, & Loeb, 2016) and providing scaffolding, which is defined as "…a form of incremental support for learners aids them in organizing and monitoring their learning, as they complete different stages in the inquiry process. The learners can then be empowered to take control of their own learning" (p. 138). Yoo and Huang (2013) explored the role of gender, age, and prior experience with online courses.

Further examination by Guan and Stanford (2016) discovered three factors that contributed to the success of online courses: institutional support for faculty, technical infrastructure, and course development. Bowen noted that "Faculty members also play a critical role in improving learner motivation and should understand that motivating students is an essential part of teaching" (as cited in Guan & Stanford, 2016). Additionally, one must consider intrinsic motivation and strive to activate and maintain it. Stephenson (2018) raises the issue of intrinsic motivation in voice students but offers no comments on how to invoke it. Thorsell (2014) identified three factors that help build intrinsic motivation: self-determination, social interaction, and the role of leaders. Thorsell (2014) further noted the role of self-determination, social interaction, and the role of leadership in student motivation. Though subtle, both extrinsic and particularly intrinsic motivation has a strong influence on student motivation. See table 4 for motivational characteristics that affect student success in online learning.

DISCUSSION

What has been learned from the literature? Regarding learner characteristics, their innate sense of isolation should be combated. Take time to screen those who plan to take online courses. Select students who have completed online courses. Promote self-efficacy among potential online students or those who are currently enrolled in courses. Seek to discover and promote motivation that works for these students. Regarding technical characteristics, select reliable and intuitive learning management systems (LMS) and provide 24/7 technical support. These actions will go far to remove technical barriers. Course designers and facilitators should recognize various barriers to learning and strive to reduce them. Incorporate the use of mobile technology as an adjunct or supplement to more standard computing systems. Regarding administrative characteristics, administrators and facilitators should promote affective learning engagement (ALE). Also, they should analyze institutional data better to understand and accommodate their student learners. To improve learning, students should be taught to use self-regulating techniques. Students should be continuously motivated throughout the life of the course. Finally,

Table 4. Motivational elements affecting student success in online learning

Characteristic(s)	Purpose
Gender	Female students seem to do better online than do male students.
Age	Though producing mixed results in various studies, it appears that older students participate more in online learning than do younger students.
Student's prior online experience	Though producing mixed results in various studies, a student's previous online experience tended to be a positive indicator of success in subsequent online courses.
Self-determination	Scheutz (as cited in Thorsell, 2014) noted that "The student self-determination theory argues, "community college students who experience a robust sense of belonging, competency, and autonomy will naturally be more engaged" (p. 79).
Social interaction	Thorsell, 2014) noted that "...connecting with others is an emotional experience. Handelsman et al. (as cited in Thorsell, 2014) concluded that emotion is one of the strongest types of student engagement and an important part of intrinsic motivation" (p. 80).
Role of leaders	Several studies (as cited in Thorsell, 2014) "...have shown that transformational leadership style generates deeper engagement in students" (p. 80).
Other factors	Online students demonstrate stronger motivation than on-campus face to face students on three intrinsic motivation scales: to know, to accomplish, and to experience stimulation (Rovai, Ponton, Wighting, and Baker, 2007).

one must have an awareness of the role of motivation, particularly intrinsic motivation, in student engagement and learning.

EXAMPLES FOR LEARNER CHARACTERISTICS

We have identified the demographics of this class, which are traditional college juniors representing African-Americans, Hispanics, and Caucasians races. Whether the class is face-to-face or online, certain factors should be considered by the teacher or facilitator.

History, Science, Literature, and Archaeology

All four examples make use of the constructivist learning theory or cognitivist learning theory. This provides a unifying thread that ties these four examples together. All these courses make use of visual material gathered from the Internet. The links to sites on the web provides visual and aural stimulation. Group work reduces isolation by having everyone assigned to one of the teams that address each objective, which is characteristic of the constructivist learning theory in which learners construct their own knowledge. Working with other students is a good way to go about achieving this through group or teamwork. The teacher or facilitator could lead the class with a transformative leadership style, which would likely provide emotional and intellectual support for students to succeed, to help motivate them, to help develop self-determination.

SUMMARY

A review of the literature, even limited to the years 2011 to 2016, revealed a significant body of research about online learner characteristics. These materials were generally in agreement with those elements that support these learners. Online learning seems to have become a permanent part of effective methods of reaching those who wish to learn in this manner. It seems that there is no longer any meaningful debate about the ability to learn from online courses. For example, Cao and Sakchutchawan (2011) concluded that faculty and employers who hold negative views of online learning have no strong foundation for such perceptions. Those students who wish to learn and apply themselves can perform very well in online courses. A different set of skills are required for online learning, but these skills are neither unobtainable nor difficult to acquire. Online learning simply requires a different mindset and a different approach. It is notable that no such effort to justify the traditional methods of imparting knowledge has ever been undertaken. Perhaps, there was little or no reason to engage in such activity in those days because there was no other way to reach students aside from face to face instruction. Looking to the future, students have additional options for engagement in learning, such as telecommunications and mobile computing technology.

Chapter 7 contains a discussion of instructional technology including portable and hand-held devices and their application to higher education. The future of instructional technology is briefly discussed as are emerging technologies. The chapter ends with a presentation of how SMART technology can be used in four major undergraduate curriculum areas.

REFERENCES

Alqurashi, E. (2016). Self-Efficacy in Online Learning Environments: A Literature Review. *Contemporary Issues in Education Research*, *9*(1), 45–52. doi:10.19030/cier.v9i1.9549

Arndt, T., & Guercio, A. (2014). Ubiquitous E-Learning: Student Attitudes and Future Prospects. *GSTF Journal on Computing*, *4*(1), 77.

Aversa, E., & MacCall, S. (2013). Profiles in retention part 1: Design characteristics of a graduate synchronous online program. *Journal of Education for Library and Information Science*, *54*(2), 147–161. Retrieved from http://search.proquest.com/docview/1399142296?accountid=35812

Bettinger, E., Liu, J., & Loeb, S. (2016). Connections matter: How interactive peers affect students in online college courses. *Journal of Policy Analysis and Management*, *35*(4), 1–25. doi:10.1002/pam.21932

Bouhnik, D., & Golan, C. (2012). E-course: ICT elements and students' thinking dispositions. *I-Manager's. Journal of Information Technology*, *1*(4), 19–34. Retrieved from http://search.proquest.com/docview/1473904448?accountid=35812

Cao, Y., & Sakchutchawan, S. (2011). Online vs. traditional MBA: An empirical study of students' characteristics, course satisfaction, and overall success. *The Journal of Human Resource and Adult Learning*, *7*(2), 1–12. Retrieved from http://search.proquest.com/docview/1016739835?accountid=35812

Centers for Disease Control and Prevention. (2013). *E-Learning Design: E-Learning Essentials*. Retrieved from http://www.cdc.gov/learning/quality/essentials.html

Choi, B. (2016). How people learn in an asynchronous online learning environment: The relationships between graduate students' learning strategies and learning satisfaction | Comment apprennent les gens dans un environnement d'apprentissage en ligne asynchrone. *Canadian Journal of Learning and Technology*, *42*(1). doi:10.21432/T24K7R

Clark, A., & Fishleigh, J. (2012), E-learning and the legal foundations course: It's (a bit of) a revolution! *Legal Information Management*, *12*, 235-238. doi:10.1017/S1472669612000527

Cortés, A., & Barberá, E. (2013). Time patterns and perceptions of online learning success factors. *eLearn Center Research Paper Series*, (7), 39-48.

Gappi, L. L. (2013). Relationships between learning style preferences and academic performance of students. *International Journal of Educational Research and Technology*, *4*(2), 70–76.

Guan, S., & Stanford, D. (2016). Learner and faculty support. *New Directions for Higher Education, 2016*(173), 65–74. doi:10.1002/he.20180

Hachey, A. C., Wladis, C. W., & Conway, K. M. (2012). Is the Second Time the Charm? Investigating Trends in Online Re-Enrollment, Retention and Success. *Journal of Educators Online*, *9*(1), n1. doi:10.9743/JEO.2012.1.2

Irby, T. L., & Strong, R. (2015). A synthesis of mobile learning research implications: Agricultural faculty and student acceptance of mobile learning in academia. *NACTA Journal*, *59*(1), 10–17. Retrieved from http://search.proquest.com/docview/1660304997?accountid=35812

Kamali, A. (2014). Attributes of Affective E-learning Behavior: Emerging Issues Beyond Teaching and Learning. *US-China Education Review*, 705.

Kianmehr, L., & Kamali, A. (2013). Correlates of Learning Behaviors and Performance Outcomes in e-Learning. In *Proceedings of the Information Systems Educators Conference* (Vol. 2167, p. 1435). Academic Press.

Kirby, D., Barbour, M. K., & Sharpe, D. B. (2015). Student Perceptions and Preferences for Tertiary Online Courses: Does Prior High School Distance Learning Make a Difference? *Education Faculty Publications*. Retrieved from http://digitalcommons.sacredheart.edu/ced_fac/114

Kruger-Ross, M. J., & Waters, R. D. (2013). Predicting online learning success: Applying the situational theory of publics to the virtual classroom. *Computers & Education*, *61*, 176-184.

Philip, K. E. J., & Lee, A. C. (2011). Online Public Health Education for Low and Middle-Income Countries: Factors Influencing Successful Student Outcomes. *International Journal of Emerging Technologies in Learning*, *6*(4), 65–69. doi:10.3991/ijet.v6i4.1797

Rovai, A. P., Ponton, M. K., Wighting, M. J., & Baker, J. D. (2007). A comparative analysis of student motivation in traditional classroom and E-learning courses. *International Journal on E-Learning*, *6*(3), 413–432. Retrieved from http://search.proquest.com/docview/210329343?accountid=35812

Salyers, V., Carter, L., Carter, A., Myers, S., & Barrett, P. (2014). The search for meaningful e-learning at Canadian universities: A multi-institutional research study. *The International Review of Research in Open and Distributed Learning*, *15*(6). doi:10.19173/irrodl.v15i6.1713

Seiver, J. G., & Troja, A. (2014). Satisfaction and Success in Online Learning as a Function of the Needs for Affiliation, Autonomy, and Mastery. *Distance Education*, *35*(1), 90–105. doi:10.1080/01587919.2014.891427

Smith, R. (2010). *Motivational factors in e-learning*. Retrieved from http://www.ruthcsmith.com/wordpress/wp-content/uploads/2012/10/Motivation.pdf

Stark, E., Lassiter, A., & Kuemper, A. (2013). A brief examination of predictors of e-learning success for novice and expert learners. *Knowledge Management & E-Learning*, *5*(3), 269–277.

Stephenson, K. (2018). Critical Thought, Intrinsic Motivation, and the Voice Studio: Perspectives of Master Teachers. *Journal of Singing: the Official Journal of the National Association of Teachers of Singing*, *74*(4), 405–414.

Thorsell, L. A. (2014). Graduate certificates in Ontario colleges: Uniquely engaging in specialized skills development. *Higher Education. Skills and Work-Based Learning*, *5*(1), 74–85. doi:10.1108/HESWBL-08-2014-0037

Wendt, J., & Wendt, S. (2012, October). Online course success: Adapting course design to focus on learning. In *Proceedings of World Conference on E-Learning in Corporate, Government, Healthcare, and Higher Education* (pp. 448-452). Academic Press.

Wladis, C., Hachey, A. C., & Conway, K. (2013). Are online students in STEM (science, technology, engineering and mathematics) courses at greater risk of non-success? *American Journal of Educational Studies*, *6*(1), 65.

Xu, D., & Jaggars, S. S. (2013). The impact of online learning on students' course outcomes: Evidence from a large community and technical college system. *Economics of Education Review*, *37*, 46–57. doi:10.1016/j.econedurev.2013.08.001

Yoo, J. Y., & Huang, W. D. (2013). Engaging online adult learners in higher education: Motivational factors impacted by gender, age, and prior experiences. *The Journal of Higher Education*, *61*(3), 151–164.

Section 3
The Future

The third of four parts concerns the future and tying the preceding chapters together. Chapter 7 contains a treatment of the ongoing evolution of instructional technology. A word of caution, however, is called for because sound pedagogical principles and activities comes before technology. Technology for the sake of technology is an unwise approach. There must be an underlying rationale and principles for applying instructional technology to pedagogy. Portable and hand-held devices receive discussion, as does the application of these devices to higher education and in the context of how the human brain operates. The next element concerns the future and emerging technologies; however, one must bear in mind the of greater precedence is information and communications technology (ICT), because ICT subsumes application of technology to teaching and learning. Chapter 8 is devoted to tying the preceding chapters together into a coherent philosophy of teaching and learning. It contains a review of the important elements in the preceding chapters. Chapter 9 is devoted to a surmise of education in the future. This includes driving forces such as occupations that are becoming obsolete and those that are arising with new technology. The subject is discussed in the context of education, politics, policy, the economy, and the environment.

Figure 1.

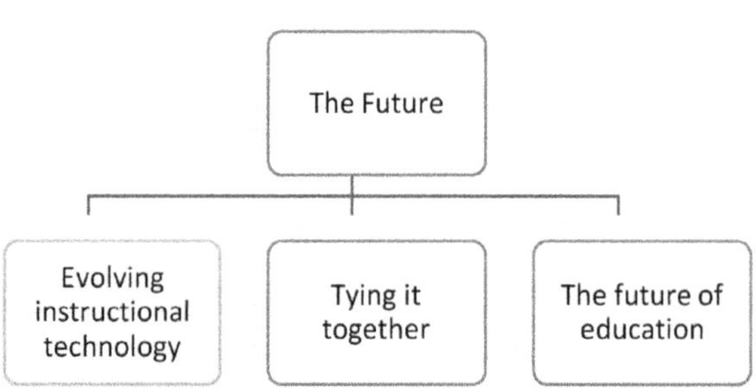

Chapter 7
Evolving Instructional Technology

ABSTRACT

Technology applied to education is developing and becoming more sophisticated at an increasingly rapid pace. Examples include both hardware and software applications among which are course materials such as those open course ware and massive online open courses. Mobile communications via portable and hand-held digital devices provide the means to acquire and interact with courses and course materials. These small devices show considerable promise for application in higher education by making a reality of learning anytime, anyplace. There are two keys to successful operation: the cloud and learning management systems (LMSs). These and yet-to-be-created technologies are making many jobs and occupations obsolete while creating new ones. This rapid change requires a new set of globally oriented people and business skills. Education systems must recognize this change and prepare students to meet the challenges. Two emerging technologies are 3-D printing and blockchain.

EVOLVING INSTRUCTIONAL TECHNOLOGY

Instructional technology is evolving along with the information explosion. The need becomes one of how to apply this technology to teaching and learning. Technology that is easy to use, ubiquitous, effective, and reliable is needed. Not being a prophet, one cannot predict the future with any degree

DOI: 10.4018/978-1-7998-1542-6.ch007

Figure 1.

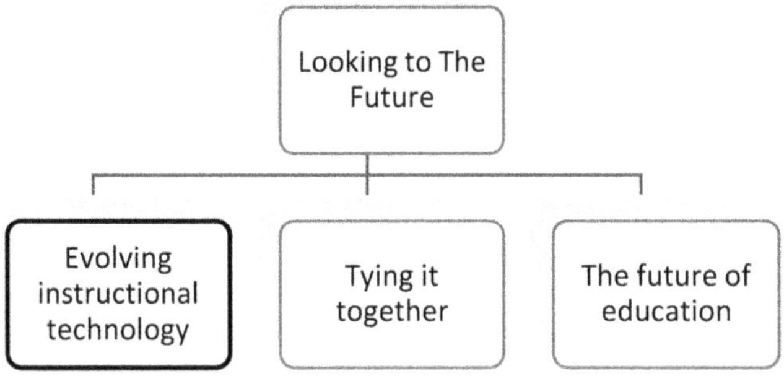

of accuracy, but the evolving role of technology can be predicted to produce as yet the undreamed-of capability to help people to learn.

Two examples are Open Course Ware (OCW) and Massive Online Open Courses (MOOC). According to "Opencourseware"(2018), OCW "are course lessons created at universities and published for free via the Internet" (para. 1). This source further states that in the latter part of the 1990s OCW projects appeared, first in Europe and later in the United States (OpenCourseWare, 2018). Educause defines a Massive Online Open Courses as "…a model for delivering learning content online to any person who wants to take a course, with no limit on attendance (Massive Open Online Course (MOOC) (n.d.), para, 1). It seems that MOOCs are a more recent innovation than OCW.

One cannot help but wonder what is the difference between the Open Course Ware and the Massive Online Open Course? To some degree, they might be synonymous. On the other hand, there does seem to be a difference. Stephan (2015) of UCI University of California Irvine makes a distinction between them. For example, Open Course Ware "…consists primarily of teaching materials used by university faculty members in teaching their regular courses supplemented by lecture videos" (para. 3). He notes that a Massive Online Open Course "…is a highly designed collection of teaching materials combined with learning assessments and (in a few cases) opportunities for students to interact with each other through discussion forums and peer-graded activities" (Stefan, para 2).

PORTABLE AND HAND-HELD DIGITAL DEVICES

This leads to a consideration of how students interact with these kinds of courses. There are, of course, PCs. A newer addition to the arsenal of learning tools is the mobile hand-held digital device. According to "Types of Handheld Devices, Handheld Device Software, Handheld Gadgets, What Are Handheld Devices"(n.d.), such an appliance

...is a pocket-sized computing device with a display screen and input/output interface like an external or touch screen keyboard. Going by this definition of handheld devices and gadgets many appliances can qualify to be called handheld, like a mobile phone, PDA, mobile PC, handheld game consoles and so on" (para. 1).

The same source lists several such devices, which include the following:

- Mobile computers
- Notebook PC
- Ultra-Mobile PC
- Handheld PC
- Personal digital assistant/Enterprise digital assistant
- Graphing calculator
- Pocket computer (largely obsolete)
- Handheld game consoles
- Nintendo DS (NDS)
- Game Boy, Game Boy Color
- Game Boy Advance
- Sega Game Gear
- PC Engine GT
- Pokémon Mini
- NeoGeo Pocket, NeoGeo Color
- Atari Lynx
- Pandora
- GP2X/GP32
- Gizmondo
- PlayStation Portable (PSP)
- N-Gage

Media recorders

- Digital still camera (DSC)
- Digital video camera (DVC or digital Camcorder)
- Digital audio recorders
- Media players/displayers
- Portable media player
- e-book reader

Communication devices

- Mobile phone
- Cordless telephone
- Pager (Types of Handheld Devices, Handheld Device Software, Handheld Gadgets, What are Handheld Devices (n.d.), para. 2).

These devices carry many benefits and are very popular such that they are readily adopted by a great many users despite age, gender, nationality, race, and ethnicity. Further, these tools make possible an office on the go, they have high convenience, they carry entertainment, and they break the communication barrier ("Types Of Handheld Devices, Handheld Device Software, Handheld Gadgets, What Are Handheld Devices", n.d.). The future is bright for these appliances.

APPLICATION TO HIGHER EDUCATION

It is not surprising that these digital, handheld devices are finding a role in education at every level, including higher education. The technical requirements include a learning management system (LMS) and a device to access the internet in the cloud on which reside these learning activities and materials. Cloud computing makes it possible to use application software that resides in the cloud rather than on each handheld device, thus lowering cost and conserving storage space on the application.

A great many apps are available for various disciplines. In fact, there are so many that it becomes increasingly difficult to keep up with them. Lynch (2017) a list such devices "…116 of the best teaching and learning apps" para. 1). Lynch (2017) goes on to say that

…students can individually learn, practice, study, and have fun with different subjects and concepts. Luckily, there are many good, quality apps for students

of all ages. It is important to note that this list is separated into categories, and the apps in each category are not in rank ordered" (para. 3).

These categories are as follows: virtual reality apps, math apps, assorted teaching-learning apps, teacher communication apps, movie-making apps, study skills apps, science apps, social studies apps, grammar and spelling skills apps, writing skills apps, and creativity apps. In Table 1 the quantity of apps within each category is listed. While these apps include primary and secondary schools, many of them would also apply to higher education.

The "Tablet Pc" (n.d.) website defines a tablet PC as a device that is

a portable PC that is a hybrid between a personal digital assistant (PDA) and notebook PC. Equipped with a touch screen interface, a tablet PC usually has a software application used to run a virtual keyboard. However, many tablet PCs support external keyboards.

Tablet PCs have built-in Web browsing capabilities, multiple connectivity options, capacitive touch screens and multimedia - including high definition (HD) support. Tablet PCs are also equipped with accelerometers, which allow users to view display screens in portrait or landscape mode (para. 1). A keyboard and mouse that can be attached are

optional, while the instrument is still considered a tablet computer. This device seems to be the best option for mobile computing because it permits the use of a keyboard and mouse to create assignments that are to be composed as formal academic documents.

Technical requirements for use in education include a learning management system (LMS) and a device that can transmit and receive data to and from the LMS. There are many devices that satisfy this requirement and a variety of learning management systems. Additionally, connection to the cloud is important because the software applications can reside in the cloud and thereby alleviate the necessity of housing these apps on the digital device. There are a host of teaching and learning apps. Lynch, M. (2017) identifies 116 of them. Table 1 lists them by types.

It is apparent that one has available all kinds of programs on which to create instructional activities. Then, there are various authoring software programs, many of which reside in the cloud. Christopher Pappas (2012) lists 50 authoring software programs, 150 learning management systems, 55 cloud-based eLearning authoring tools, 20 cloud-based LMSs, and so on (Pappas, 2012). A learning management system is defined as

Table 1. The number of applications

Category	Number of Apps
Virtual reality	20
Math	23
Assorted teaching and learning	17
Teacher communication	2
Movie making	5
Study Skills	3
Science	10
Social studies	10
Grammar and Spelling	4
Writing skills	6
Creativity	16
Total	116
Adapted from Lynch (2017).	

a software application or Web-based technology used to plan, implement, and assess a specific learning process. Typically, a learning management system provides an instructor with a way to create and deliver content, monitor student participation, and assess student performance. A learning management system may also provide students with the ability to use interactive features such as threaded discussions, video conferencing, and discussion forums (Rouse, n.d., para. 1).

Learning management systems coupled with authoring software programs, cloud-based computing, and cloud-based learning management systems hold considerable promise for use of educational technology both now and in the future.

THE FUTURE

The future remains a great unknown, but one can make guesses about instructional technology, teaching, and learning as it may exist in the future. New technologies promise to make it easier and faster for students. As Kali B (2019) put it "New technologies promise to make it easier and faster for students to learn" (para. 2). Most educators feel that traditional textbooks will be replaced by digital textbooks. Virtual reality is emerging, as is gamification in which students are enticed to complete school work to rise to higher levels. Online programs are growing and will continue to grow. These various resources are not only for the K-12 environment, but they are also being used and will be used in higher education.

Career fields are rapidly changing. Many of today's occupations develop, flourish, and disappear in a short span of time. In some cases, a profession for which one is preparing upon entering college can disappear by the time he or she graduates. For example, a Navy radio operator (Radioman 2nd class) was discharged in October of 1969. By 1997 this rating was discontinued. Morse code is no longer taught in any of the military branches including the U. S. Coast Guard. Satellite communications and computers have largely taken on communication responsibilities. This is not the only occupation that was affected by growing technology. For example, there are no longer any occupations for telephone operators, typists, and so forth. The growth of the interstate highway system and the advent of the diesel locomotive brought about the decline of the railroad industry. The question becomes the following: What does the future hold for career preparation?

Rouhiainen (2019) shares his views on what he thinks will be the primary skills of successfully educated persons. These fall into two areas: people skills and business skills. Among the people skills are self-awareness and self-assessment. He has his students engage in a personal SWOT (strengths, weaknesses, opportunities, and threats) analysis, which has proved very popular with them. Next is emotional intelligence, which he defines as "...one's capacity to be aware of and express emotions" (p. 73). Next is interpersonal intelligence. This people skill is followed by empathy and active listening. Cultural flexibility is the next one, which is followed by perseverance and passion. Then, there is a focus on the common good. Mindfulness and meditation come next. Physical training and storytelling end the list of people skills. See table 2 for more.

Business skills for the future (Rouhiainen, 2019) include those listed in Table 3. Problem-solving heads the list. Creativity and adaptability to new technology make an appearance. An entrepreneurial mindset follows. Next, are sales and marketing skills. Data analysis is a must. Presentation skills follow. Environmental intelligence is becoming increasingly important. Large scale thinking becomes more vital as the world becomes more and more globalized. Accounting and money management is necessary for success in the future world. Despite or in spite of all-encompassing technology, it is essential to unplug. Spotting trends become more and more important in the

Table 2. People skills for the future

Skill	Explanation
Self-awareness and Self-assessment	It helps people to recognize the full potential and areas that could benefit from improvement.
Emotional intelligence	As the business world becomes more complex, persons with high emotional intelligence will likely get ahead faster.
Social intelligence	Learning to understand how to work with others becomes increasingly important.
Interpersonal intelligence	Recognizing the value of personal interactions with others, particularly family, friends, and colleagues in the face of growing technology will become increasingly important.
Empathy and active listening	Exercising patience and demonstrating our valuing of another person's perspective will help us to gain insight.
Cultural flexibility	To adapt to new cultures is more and more important in the age of globalization.
Perseverance and passion	This is a primary predictor of success.
Focus on the common good	We need to go beyond thinking only of ourselves and think of what is good for everyone.
Mindfulness and meditation	These activities are vital to our wellbeing and effectiveness. Steve Jobs of Apple Computer practiced these skills.
Physical training	It is particularly important for good brain function to engage in physical activity.
Storytelling	People have always and will probably continue to thrive on storytelling. This is the ability to present one's message in story form.

Table created from material by Rouhiainen (2019) pp.71-76

context of the exponential growth of technology offers opportunities to take advantage of it. Design thinking and design mindset will help the persons having this skill to find solutions to problems that we cannot even imagine today. See table 3 for more.

EMERGING TECHNOLOGIES

Two emerging technologies with respect to education are 3-D printing and blockchain technology, which is used to authenticate certificates. Rouhiainen (2019) notes that "…3-D printing means that you can take any digital file and turn it into a three-dimensional physical object" (p. 84). Rouhiainen defines blockchain technology as a "block of chains that is used to record transactions" (p. 84). Such transactions in education can be used to track academic achievements.

Table 3. Business skills for the future

Skill	Explanation
Problem-solving	As the speed, technological innovations accelerate and the changing way in which people do business the skills become increasingly important.
Creativity	It becomes increasingly important for persons to develop unique and innovative ways to introduce new technology.
Adaptability to new technology	In addition to showing students lead the pack in new technologies, they should be taught about creative ways to put this technology to work in the classroom.
Entrepreneurial mindset	As technological innovations emerge, people should be aware of how to apply them.
Sales and marketing	These are particularly important for students who may at some point in the future to start their own businesses.
Data analysis	The enhanced capabilities of artificial intelligence and the emergence of new technologies the need to analyze data effectively will become a primary tool.
Presentation skills	It is important for educators to develop strong presentation skills, both personally and digitally. As always, it is highly important to inspire and motivate others.
Environmental intelligence	The value of preserving resources is becoming more and more apparent.
Large-scale thinking	As globalization increases, so will the need for thinking about and analyzing large organizations.
Design thinking and design mindset	With the advent of new products and services will come the need for solving problems that arise from them.

Table created from material by Rouhiainen (2019) pp.76-84

Three-Dimensional Printing

Three-dimensional (3-D) printing is rapidly growing and becoming more popular in education. TeachThought Staff (2015) identifies 10 ways in which 3-D printing can be used in education:

1. Engineering design students can print out prototypes
2. Architecture students can print out 3D models of designs
3. History classes can print out historical artifacts for examination
4. Graphic Design students can print out 3D versions of their artwork
5. Geography students can print out topography, demographic, or population maps
6. Cooking students can create molds for food products
7. Automotive students can print out replacement parts or modified examples of existing parts for testing

8. Chemistry students can print out 3D models of molecules
9. Biology students can print out cells, viruses, organs, and other critical biological artifacts
10. Math students can print out "problems" to solve in their own learning spaces, from scale models to city infrastructural design challenges (para. 6).

There is no doubt many other ways in which 3-D printing will likely be used in higher education.

Blockchain Technology

Blockchain technology can be used to virtually eliminate fraudulent credentials in higher education. First, a description of blockchain technology is necessary. For example, consider a bank and the many transactions that it experiences each day. A record of these transactions is kept in the bank's ledger. In blockchain technology, there are many units that record this information other than the bank. These discrete units are tied together in such a way to make it extraordinarily difficult or impossible for anyone to manipulate the data. This approach was limited initially to financial transactions, an example of which is bitcoin. However, it can be used in many other situations including higher education. See table 4 for more information.

EXAMPLES OF HOW SMART TECHNOLOGY CAN BE USED

History

Providing links via learning management systems to appropriate websites that students can access via handheld or portable computing devices will be one use of SMART technology. These could be links to the music of the period for students to analyze the lyrics. Hearing the authentic Rebel Yell and its use as a psychological weapon. Reading first-person accounts of how Southerners experienced Sherman's March to the Sea. Excerpts from books can be used to expand on the topic. All these resources among others can help today's students to empathize with the feelings held by participants in that great struggle. Instructional technology can easily provide excerpts

Table 4. Blockchain technology applied to higher education

Use	Explanation
1. Using a blockchain for automatic recognition and transfer of credits	Eases the complexity and burden of accurately transferring academic credits.
2. Blockchains for tracking intellectual property and rewarding use and re-use of that property	Accurate tracking and sharing of knowledge without restrictions.
3. Using verified sovereign identities for student identification within educational organizations	Reduces the risk of unintentional disclosure of personal information identification.
4. Using a blockchain as a lifelong learning passport	A digitally "verifiable CV" would limit credential fraud, and significantly reduce organizational workload in credential verification.
5. Using blockchains to permanently secure certificates	Reduces the expense and burden of obtaining and forwarding transcripts.
6. Using blockchains to verify multi-step accreditation	To check and verify the accuracy of accreditation.

This table was compiled from data from Yardy (2018).

from Ken Burn's *The Civil War* series. This technology can make it possible for students to form groups via the Internet to complete assignments and otherwise work together on teams. Anytime, anywhere learning could be made available for students via iPads and similar devices that they could use in odd moments of free time such as on breaks at work, traveling on buses or commuter trains, and during any other snatches of time, they might find. Furthermore, the brain likes this kind of brief but intensive exposure to the learning material. A compatible LMS and the cloud would make devices with modest memories and capacities function in a highly sophisticated manner. A virtual field trip to some of the museums in Washington, D.C. and other places concerning the War Between the States could be assigned.

Science

Even modest instructional technology can provide students access to sites on the web that have footage of fluorescing calcium ions thus making cardiac cellular electrical activity visible. Links can be provided to sites that have footage showing time-lapse photography of nerve cells migrating to join with similar-minded nerve cells. Animations that show action potentials as they fire to generate electrical flow along neurons, some of which extend all the way from the spine to the foot. Via this technology students have the means of interacting in groups when they are separated by distance, through software such as Skype. The cloud can be used to access word processing software and other apps like PowerPoint and Excel to create dynamic reports.

An appropriate LMS and data and app storage on the cloud would make these snippets of instruction available over small, digital hand-held devices.

Literature

Make links to archival recordings of folk music and ballads from performers of years ago. They could use apps like Nvivo to transcribe the lyrics and analyze their content. By use of appropriate software on the cloud, students could write the results of their analyses and illustrate the report with graphs, photographic images, and other materials necessary to give the narratives life. There could also be links to sites featuring famous authors such as Washington Irving, Nathaniel Hawthorne, and others who used themes from folklore. All of this could be made possible by way of the cloud, a good LMS, and a hand-held digital device. Such a device and communications and data storage system could prove to be powerful learning tools, but a composition of formal papers on these small devices would prove to be excessively time-consuming without a keyboard input; therefore, there would also be a need for students to have access to such apps to compose formal academic documents.

Archaeology

The nature of archaeology has changed with advancing technology. Links could be provided for sites such as Google Earth for students to study terrain for signs of ancient settlements. Ground-penetrating radar helps archaeologists see beneath the earth for evidence of artifacts of ancient civilizations. Lidar is used to strip away jungle growth and thus unveil lost cities in Central America and in other parts of the world. Side scanning sonar is helpful to locate underwater ruins. All this technology is making learning more and more exciting, efficient, and effective. Authoring software programs can be used to simulate all manner of interactions with students. It is now possible to apply all the nine events of instruction via these devices that were identified by Dr. Robert Gagné (1985), particularly, providing learner guidance and giving feedback via the features of these programs. Artificial intelligence will play an increasingly significant role in evolving instructional technology. The TeachThought Staff (2018) website offers 10 roles for artificial intelligence in education: 1) automate routine repetitive activities such as grading, 2) adapt educational software to student needs, 3) identify places for improvement in courses, 4) help for students by artificial intelligence tutors, 5) provide teachers and students with helpful feedback, 6) altering how we find and interact with information, 7) could change the role of teachers, 8) make trial and error learning less daunting, 9) provide data to help find, teach, and support students, 10) may change where students learn, who teaches them, and how they acquire basic skills.

APPS APPLIED TO HIGHER EDUCATION

Many, if not all, of these apps, can be applied to higher education. Among these are webinars. Though synchronous, webinars are an excellent way to bring experts and learners together. Further, these webinars can be and most often are recorded for later viewing by those who were unable to attend the event as it was unfolding, or for review by those who did attend. Webinar technology and use are descended from Live Virtual Classroom (LVC) technology and use. It does, however, rely upon a set of skills that is different from other forms of eLearning to be effective (Driscoll & Carliner, 2005). Tutorials are like webinars but are also different because a tutorial is an exchange between, typically, two individuals (the mentor and the mentee) while the webinar is an exchange between groups of persons (presenters and attendees). A tutorial can be either synchronous or asynchronous or a combination of both. E-books are another field suitable for development. These books have many features bestowed on them by the nature of this software. For example, one can highlight germane quotations and items of interest. One can copy material directly from the e-book and paste it into a document or a visual program (with proper citation, of course). In kindle, one can create a notebook from highlighted material that can be turned into flashcards for study or exported for use elsewhere. Online learning is perhaps the primary reason for using this technology. This kind of learning can be either informal or formal, depending on how it is designed and how it is used. Formal learning leads to course credit and ultimately to either degrees or certification. Informal learning leads to equipping a seeker to perform a task, such as repairing a faucet in a sink. Working on teams is another feature of how instructional technology can be used in education. In such settings, team members work together to solve problems, complete assignments, and otherwise attack tasks. Teamwork is becoming increasingly important in the corporate world, as well. With online collaboration participants can work together no matter where they are in the world (if they have internet access). These meetings can be both asynchronous and synchronous, depending on the nature of their work. Self-assessment is another feature made easy by way of online access. These assessments can range from aptitude tests to tests over the subject matter. One tremendous advantage of online self-assessment is the speed with which the results of these tests are returned. This is an important feature because immediate feedback is a powerful learning tool. Blending artificial intelligence with this function can produce highly personalized reviews.

M-learning (mobile learning) can make learning anywhere, anytime a reality. Short podcasts over specific subject matter make it easier for learners to acquire, use, and remember information. Driscoll and Carliner (2005) provide an example of providing product information to salespersons on the floor of department stores in very short "alerts" that are like text messages in that they are short and contain only relevant material.

SUMMARY

Instructional technology is certainly evolving and growing. Open Course Ware (OCW) and Massive Open Online Courses (MOOC) are but two examples of the democratization of education that is taking place. Through these two movements, well-known universities are creating courses and offering them to the world at large and at no cost. Handheld digital devices are increasing in number and sophistication. These devices are making learning any time anywhere practical and effective, permitting students to grab bits of free time to engage in their course work. In fact, the brain likes this approach of using snippets of information to avoid the straying of one's attention, as neuroscientists are discovering. The vast array of handheld and portable computing appliances are making a positive impact on higher education. It is very likely that the education of tomorrow will bear little resemblance to the education of yesteryear.

In chapter 8, the preceding chapters of the book are tied together. The topics include communication with the outside world, memory formation, theories of learning, instructional design theories and models, learner characteristics, and evolving instructional technology. The chapter ends with a discussion of how evolving technology can be used in four academic undergraduate programs. Chapter 9 a look at the future of education is attempted.

REFERENCES

B, K. (2019). *The future of education and technology*. Retrieved from https://elearningindustry.com/future-of-education-and-technology

Driscoll, M., & Carliner, S. (2005). *Advanced web-based training strategies: Unlocking instructionally sound online learning*. San Francisco, CA: Pfeiffer.

Lynch, M. (2017). *The tech edvocate's 2018 list of 116 of the best teaching and learning apps*. Retrieved from https://www.thetechedvocate.org/tech-edvocates-2017-list-116-best-teaching-learning-apps/

OpenCourseWare. (2018). Retrieved from https://en.wikipedia.org/wiki/OpenCourseWare

Pappas, C. (2012). *List of authoring tools: Part 1*. Retrieved from https://elearningindustry.com/list-of-authoring-tools-part-1

Rouhiainen, L. (2019). The future of higher education: How emerging technologies will change education forever. *Kindle*. Retrieved from amazon.com

Rouse, M. (n.d.). *Learning management system (LMS)*. Retrieved from https://searchcio.techtarget.com/definition/learning-management-system

Stefan, M. S. (2015). *MOOC? OCW? Which one?* Retrieved from https://sites.uci.edu/opencourseware/blog/2015/10/02/mooc-ocw-which-one/

TabletP. C. (n.d.). Retrieved from https://www.techopedia.com/definition/2662/tablet-pc

TeachThought Staff. (2015). *10 Ways 3D printing can be used In education* [infographic]. Retrieved from https://www.teachthought.com/technology/10-ways-3d-printing-can-be-used-in-education/

Types of Handheld Devices, Handheld Device Software, Handheld Gadgets, What are Handheld Devices. (n.d.). Retrieved from https://www.roseindia.net/services/mobile/What-are-Handheld-Devices.shtml

Yardy, D. (2018). *Blockchain in brief: Six ways it can transform higher education*. Retrieved from https://www.eab.com/blogs/it-forum-perspectives/2018/01/blockchain-higher-education-uses

Chapter 8
Tying it Together

ABSTRACT

Here, the proposed conceptual framework is brought together as a whole. It begins with the way we communicate with and know the external world by way of our five senses. The roles of the emotions in the memory are examined as memory is foundational to learning. Theories of learning play an important role in the conceptual framework. From the multitude of those available, we must select one or parts of several to apply to the task. One must also consider the various instructional design models and theories and select the one that best fits our instructional objectives. The nine instructional events as identified by Dr. Robert Gagné serves as a pattern for delivering instruction. Learner characteristics provide insight on how to deliver the instruction to a group of students. Evolving instructional technology can help by providing the means of effective and efficient delivery of instruction.

TYING IT TOGETHER

Thus far, the concern has been with the discrete elements that make up the conceptual framework. The attempt in this chapter is to bring it together into a connected whole. It begins with the information explosion and the need to transform this overwhelming amount of information into knowledge. There is the danger of being swamped by all this data, this information (See figure 2 in chapter 1). Lives are so sped up that in the span of one person's life he or she may expect to have experienced several careers instead of one. It is far different from what one remembers from a childhood lived in the rural

DOI: 10.4018/978-1-7998-1542-6.ch008

Figure 1.

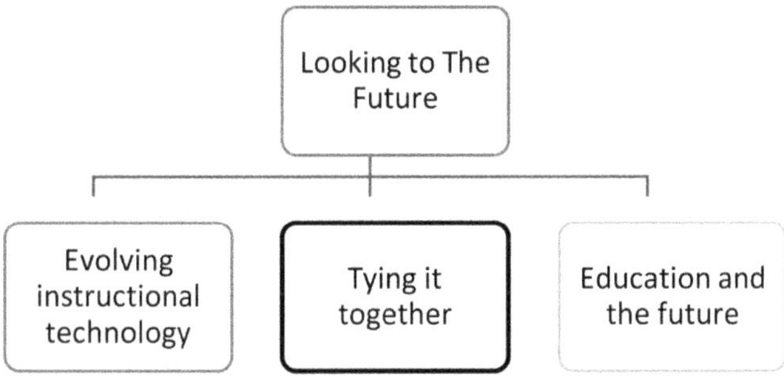

South: no electricity for rural homes, no indoor plumbing, plowing fields with a mule pulling the plow, hitching a ride on a mule-drawn wagon, though in the 1940s, the way of life was that of at least a century earlier. Information is expected to double every 12 hours, while minds are relatively static. How can one keep up with it? How can one manage this? A new view of the nature and purpose of education must be formed, and advantage of instructional technology must be taken, and this technology must be applied in ways that exploit the growing knowledge of how the brain operates.

The process for building this conceptual framework is depicted in figure 2. One must consider the subject, the objectives, the learner, the time allotted for instruction, and the resources needed to deliver the instruction. All these elements interact such that if a change is made in one box all other boxes can be affected. Based on these elements, attention can be directed to deciding on an instructional design model and a learning theory. Once done, the process of preparing the instruction for delivery must begin.

COMMUNICATION WITH THE EXTERNAL WORLD

The brain is a marvelous organ. What is known of the world is derived from sensory input, which includes smell, taste, touch, sound, and sight, all of which are transformed into electrical impulses. Transduction is the process by which this transformation from mechanical or chemical energy to electrical energy is achieved. These signals are routed to various areas of the brain where they are cataloged and processed via action potentials flowing along

Figure 2. The process for creating an instructional event

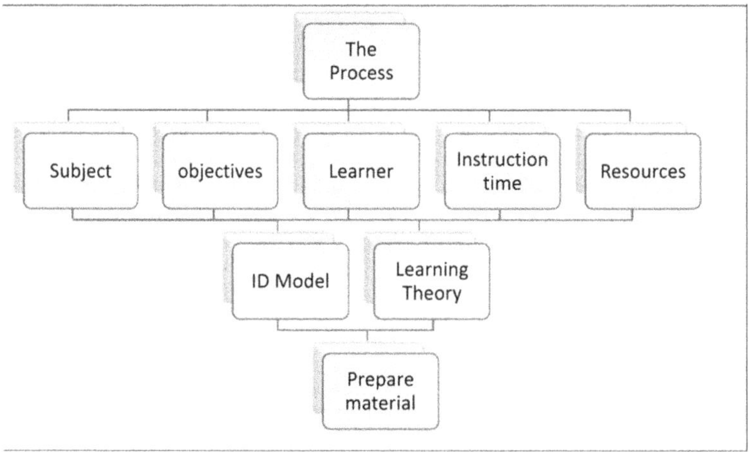

axons over synaptic space to dendrites and on to their destination. It must be recognized that what the senses perceive is limited.

For example, human visual capacity is limited to that which falls between the ultraviolent at the upper end and the infrared at the lower end of the visual spectrum. On the electromagnetic frequency spectrum, those things that one cannot see on the upper end goes on to gamma rays and on the lower end to extremely low frequency. These unseen elements far exceed what one can see in the visible spectrum. It must also be considered that fast-moving objects are not registered visually, such as bullets for example. The conclusion is that there is much more that we do not see than what we do see. Some animals, however, have a greater visual range than do humans. Our hearing capacity is also limited to between 16 Hz and 20,000 Hz (Despopoulos & Silbernagle, 1983). Dogs, bats, dolphins, and many other creatures can hear far above the human range of perception of sound. It could also be ventured to suggest that the other senses are likely as equally limited in what they can perceive. This opens the door to speculation and science fiction and the world of fantasy. There could be entire universes present around us that the senses cannot perceive. Some progress has been made with telescopes, television, telephone, microscopes and such like to expand the ability to see and hear; nevertheless, human senses are severely limited in what can be perceived, which is likely very fortunate because one might be driven mad by so much sensory input.

The emotions have a powerful influence on the expediency with which the various impulses are routed. The brain is structured so that fear or fight or flight tendency is given high priority because it could be a matter of survival.

The sense of smell is close to the limbic system (which controls human emotions) and, therefore, can have strong emotional connotations. Positive or negative traumatic events accompanied by heavy emotional content can become entrenched in memory and can be evoked during experiencing similar emotions. For example, consider the veterans who suffer Post Traumatic Stress Disorder (PTSD). Many soldiers suffered from this condition after their service to the Confederacy and the Union during the American Civil War and in previous conflicts, but this malady had no formal name at that time.

MEMORY FORMATION

Fundamental to learning is memory. There are three kinds of memory: sensory, short-term, and long-term. Sensory memory is of the shortest duration, barely achieving consciousness. If something catches one's attention, the sensation is moved to short-term memory. If the impression is of enough power, it goes to long-term memory. Fundamentally, short-term memory is just that—short term, lasting from perhaps a minute to a few minutes. Short-term memory is part of working memory. Working memory has various controls that let us manipulate the contents of short-term memory. Even so, the capacity of working memory is rather small. It can handle seven plus or minus two elements (Miller, 1994). For example, this situation in part explains why a telephone number consists of seven digits. Schemata can be formed to over overcome this shortcoming. These schemata combine these elements into concepts and such like. Schemata can be chunked together into a single concept and thereby become one unit instead of many units. Returning to the telephone number example, consider the 1-800 prefix for commercial entities. The 1-800 becomes a schema that prefixes a telephone number. Words form another example. Words are made of letters; consequently, the word becomes a schema. The formation of schemata is such that it gives great capacity to our memory and our ability to handle complex concepts consisting of many schemata. Even though our capacity consists of seven plus or minus two units of information, we can handle seven plus or minus two schemata. These schemata can be combined into yet other schemata, thus making our ability to store and retrieve information in and from our long-term memory practically infinite.

Now, turn attention to how memories are formed. It is generally agreed that neural pathways influence memory. Actions that stimulate repeated use of these pathways tend to strengthen them and the subsequent memory that they generate. It is like a path through the woods: the more it is used the stronger the trace becomes until the path becomes permanent such as with the old Native American trails, many of which became parts of major highways in modern times. Memories reside in different parts of the brain. There are many elements of memory. Imagine the first time one heard a jet airplane. It was in late summer on a beautiful afternoon. In those days, enterprising individuals (one of whom were Mr. and Mrs. Robinson) would travel around to visit small towns and villages to show movies in big tents for an entrance fee. His mother and he were visiting with the wife of this traveling movie presenter in their trailer. Then, there was this roaring sound. It was frightening, but Mrs. Robinson was unfazed. She told them it was one of these new airplanes called a jet. This memory consisted of sounds, sights, words, the feel of the dirt under the child's bare feet and other impressions. The sights are contained in the part of the brain that contains these visual images. The sounds reside in the brain where these sonic images reside. Each sensory element resides in a different place. When we recall various memories, another part of the brain coordinates the assembly of these discrete elements and synchronizes them. The amygdala, strongly associated with emotions, is included in this assembly.

One remembers similar events that have stayed with him for his entire life. One of these was a kite; the first one he had ever seen. It was a frightening image in the sky south of his boyhood home. The black diamond thrashing about in the spring sky with its knotted tail wildly flailing about in the sky. He thought it was the devil and ran into the house crying for his mother. Another such event was the play of light from a high-powered searchlight reflecting off the clouds in the night time winter sky. It looked to him like a giant illuminated hand opening and closing, grasping for something that it could not obtain. It was equally frightening. He recalls seeing the movie *Frankenstein* for the first time in the tent show owned by the Robinsons. When the electricity began whizzing and sparking during the storm in which the monster was brought to life, he and half the audience hit the ground and peered from behind the benches on which we were beforehand seated.

Now, it is time to consider how memories are retrieved from long-term memory. To begin with, something must trigger the memory. This can be an event that parallels the circumstances under which the memory was formed, a thought, or a conscious effort to recall. Such triggers can be an odor such as a fragrance associated with someone one is remembering. It could be a song or some other sound that reminds one of a past event. Once triggered, the memory can be retrieved and brought to the conscious or aware mind.

This memory, however, could have changed over time owing to the brain playing tricks on us caused by neurogenesis that created new cells to replace the old and dying ones.

THEORIES OF LEARNING

Theories of learning abound. There are nearly 100 of them. One might ask why this is the case. It seems that these theories have a certain amount of bias built into them by their creators. These theories are also the product of various degrees of experimentation. Out of this multiplicity of learning theories are four basic ones: behaviorist, cognitivist, constructivist, and connectivist. The following two books are recommended for your attention: David, L. (2017). Learning theories in plain English volumes one and two. You can find both volumes at https://www.learning-theories.com/.

The selection of a learning theory to use with the development of the material to teach should be considered. The objectives of the instruction must be well-thought-out. For example, the age of the learner, the nature of the subject, the time available for instruction, and the degree of interest that one's learners might have in the subject should be considered. The objectives concern what the subject matter is. The subject matter can cover just about anything college and university students' study: it is quite broad. The age of the learner is quite important. In higher education this can cover a spectrum spanning a range of ages and experiences from traditional freshmen to non-traditional adult learners. Next, consider the nature of the subject. Is it highly complex with definite procedures and content such as what may be encountered in science, technology, engineering, and math (STEM) topics? An additional consideration concerns the amount of time that is available for instruction. Is it a full course? A unit within a course? Does it support group work? A final consideration and vital one concerns the level of interest your learners may have in the subject. If there is little interest, they will not remember much of what they are supposed to learn. If there is high interest, half the battle is won.

People may recall the days in their classrooms. The areas that may be remembered include:Off the topic tales, stories, and anecdotes that their professors shared. For example, there was a philosophy professor who was blind in one eye. To pass the eye exam for his driver's license, he memorized the chart beforehand. Covering the bad eye, he read it off without error; covering the good eye, he repeated the performance and got the driver's license.

INSTRUCTIONAL DESIGN THEORIES AND MODELS

Closely tied to learning theories are instructional design theories and models. Two of the most common are the ADDIE model (see figure 3) and Gagné's nine instructional events (see figure 4). ADDIE is an acronym that stands for Analyze, Design, Develop, Implement, and Evaluate. Note that evaluate concerns each stage in the model. This model, like most instructional design models, is highly iterative.

The analysis is primarily of learner characteristics. One must know something about the nature of those who are to be instructed. Once analyzed, the instructional event is designed. Once designed, it is developed. Then the program is implemented. Ideally, the initial implementation would be as a beta test so that weaknesses could be identified and corrected before widespread distribution.

The nine instructional events were the creation of Dr. Robert Gagné (1985). This constitutes both a theory and a model. As depicted in figure 4, the nine events divide neatly into three stages: preparation, instruction and

Figure 3. The ADDIE model

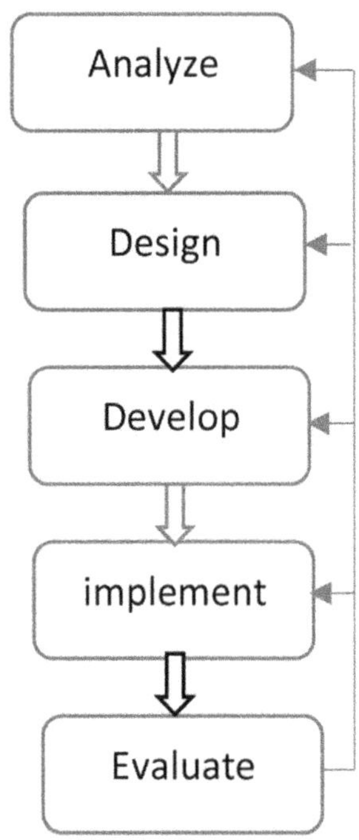

Figure 4. Gagne's nine instructional events in three phases

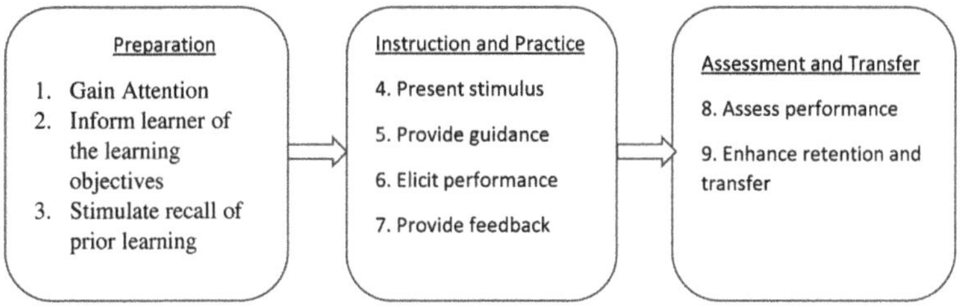

practice, and assessment and transfer. This model is more closely aligned with the method of instruction.

The preparation stage consists of gaining the attention of the audience, which could be little more than a question, or something that could be posed in a short video clip. Next would be telling learners what they will be expected to learn from the instruction and the conditions under which they would demonstrate what was learned. The final step in the preparation stage would be stimulating the learners to recall something that they already know and applying it to what they are to learn.

The instruction and practice stage is where the content of the lesson is delivered. The learning content provides a stimulus for the learner. For example, were this to use a behaviorist approach, the stimulus would be presented in small bites (programmed instruction) with guidance provided for each step. After presenting the learner with enough content to warrant his or her application of it, the learners are required to perform the behavior identified in the learning objective for this lesson. Feedback is applied as necessary to ensure that the learner has grasped and can use the new knowledge. But the key to the entire process lies in your learner characteristics.

LEARNER CHARACTERISTICS

Learner characteristics must be taken into consideration. The purpose is to present your material in a way that matches the personalities and needs of your target audience. Many have found it helpful to create an avatar or stereotype of the ideal learner that contains most of the characteristics of the target group and direct the designing and teaching to that composite individual.

EVOLVING INSTRUCTIONAL TECHNOLOGY

To make the most of the brain's idiosyncrasies, instructional technology that appeals to as many senses as possible should be used. At present this use in education amounts primarily to hearing and seeing. When these two are synchronized, a person can process up to one million bits per second as opposed to seven bits per second when listening and 50 bits per second when reading: Seeing and hearing together make a profound difference in increased capacity for the intake of information (Despopoulos & Silbernagle, 1983).

How student attention to instruction be encouraged? There are several ways: appealing to the senses, stimulating curiosity, involving the emotions. All of these are needed to meet the demands of the "new" student. Stimulating curiosity can be as simple as asking an intriguing question. Once stimulated, it must be cultivated. In short, the instructor must make the instruction interesting.

How can an emotional connection between the student and the material that he or she is learning be established? This can be and is quite difficult. Music is one way to do this, but one must be careful because musical tastes differ. Even so, the use of major and minor keys and matching tempo can extend across cultures and generation divides (Hunter, Schellenberg, & Schimmack, 2010, February). Consider one listening to Tom Roush who can be found at www.youtube.com/user/MusicOfTomRoush. Mr. Roush specializes in American music of the 19th century. He accompanies some of his music with early photographs (daguerreotypes, tintypes, carte de vistes and so forth). For example, with the song *Lorena* and other pieces as well, the music plays, and the song sung as images of attractive young women are featured in the slide show. It leaves one with a feeling of poignancy, loss, and sadness for those lovely ladies who are now dead and turned to dust as are the young men whom they loved and who died untimely deaths. It can take quite a bit of ingenuity to manipulate emotions to strengthen learning, but it can be done and done effectively.

EXAMPLES APPLIED TO EVOLVING TECHNOLOGY

Evolving technology can be applied to the examples of instructional units for history, science, literature, and archaeology. To make these units available for learners in any format, this material shall be housed in the cloud, authoring software (a class of software that makes it possible to create interaction between a learner and his or her computer) that is available in the cloud could be used to make the material interactive, and a cloud-based learning management system can be used to tie these elements together as well as providing course management features. These steps will ensure that the material is accessible to everyone with a compatible digital device ranging from standard PCs to laptop computers, and various hand-held devices which will allow users (students) to view, hear, interact with, learn, and remember while having a free moment in which to engage with the learning material.

History

The content to be delivered to the students could be arranged as a series of minilessons, that fulfill the nine instructional events of Dr. Gagné. Unlike the classroom version, this would use another learning theory, such as cognitivist. This could begin with a link to Tom Roush performing the song *Lorena* (https://www.youtube.com/watch?v=7U4yAXM53mI). This would get the viewer's attention. The song is accompanied by old photographic images of young ladies of that period of history. This captures the essence of the tragic consequences of that conflict for both the North and South. This performance is close to how it would have been performed at that time in history. Memoires of a member of Company F of the 45th Georgia Infantry wrote that "of the 125 men from Jones [County] I believe 90 of them could play the fiddle…" (S. H. Griswold cited in Williams, 2003. p. 517).

The bandwidth of this instructional sequence should be easily handled by most if not all computing devices. The objectives could be either put in text alone, or spoken by the narrator, or perhaps both. Recall of prior learning could be simply noted by a voice-over. Presentation of the learning stimulus consumes the bulk of the lesson. This could be handled by sharing links to appropriate resources and tied together with voice over. Learning guidance could be provided in an interaction point at which the learner would respond with his or her digital device to a series of prompts. Depending upon the responses, the learner would advance to another interaction point of new material in the event of a correct response, or to a remediation screen in the event of an incorrect response. Performance could be elicited through a series of screens that branch on the foundation of correct or incorrect responses. During this section, feedback could be provided to both correct and incorrect responses. Upon finishing the lesson, a short multiple-choice quiz could be presented and graded with the results immediately returned to the learner. The lesson could end with a narration summing up the nature of the material presented in the lesson and presentation of a moral to help students remember the lesson and what they learned in it. For example, "It would have been wonderful if a peaceful conclusion of the slavery issue could have been reached similar to that which occurred in England in 1833 under the driving force of Wilbur Wilberforce, but tempers flared on both sides and war was inevitable."

Science

This lesson, unlike the classroom version, would work well as either a cognitivist or a behaviorist driven presentation. If the behaviorist view were to be used, it would respond well in the form of programmed instruction in which small snippets of information are provided and followed immediately with interaction points. Using the Gagné model, the unit could begin with a link to video depicting signaling calcium ions that make electrical activity visible. This could be accompanied by a narrator saying, "Electrical activity is a vital component of life. This activity causes muscles to contract that for example keep one's heart beating." The objectives would be presented immediately following the attention-getting opening. To stimulate recall of existing knowledge, the narrator state that "This is the same principle as that which operates our computers, cell phones, air conditioners, refrigerators. The major difference lies in how the electrical current is generated and distributed." The next step is the content of the lesson which could be presented as programmed instruction. This step would be the longest of the teaching episodes. Learner guidance would be provided via branching screens the route of which would be determined by either correct or incorrect responses during presentation of the stimulus. This could be followed by a short multiple-choice quiz, the results of which could be delivered immediately upon completing the examination. Enhancing retention and recall could be strengthened by a quick review and presenting a moral to the material such as "Our bodies generate considerable electrical activity as a routine matter. The brain accounts for about 30% of this activity. So, as you go about your daily activities think about how this electricity governs the functioning of our bodies."

Literature

This lesson would also use a different learning theory from that used in the classroom because students would be expected to work in isolation of one another and participating in short snippets of time. The cognitivist or behaviorist theory could be used instead of the constructivist. To gain attention, the unit could begin with a performance of the ballad *Scarboro Fair* with a link to a performance by Simon and Garfunkel on YouTube. The objectives would be shared immediately upon the conclusion of the ballad. Recall of prior learning could be included by a narrator, who says something like the following: "In earlier times, events both large and small were captured in song. In this case, the singer recalls a love of some years past in the town of Scarboro in Yorkshire, England. Think about the songs of an earlier time and the story that the lyrics tell." The content of the lesson is presented next. This could be presented by topic with time allowed for reflection on the material, which strengthens its power in our memory. Performance could be elicited by having students create a short journal containing what they have learned from the instruction. The teacher could provide feedback on these short journal entries. The student's performance could be assessed via a short multiple-choice test the results of which could be returned immediately upon having submitted the test. Recall and retention could be stimulated by presenting a moral to the unit. The narrator could deliver such lines as these: "Folk tales and ballads tell of sad and joyous and humorous events, not unlike the news media does today. As you view a news broadcast or read it on the internet, think about how some of these stories could be immortalized in either song, tales, or both."

Archaeology

This topic could be effectively handled with programmed instruction. To get attention, route the learner to a link that shows LIDAR peeling away obscuring jungle to reveal a lost city in Central America. Follow this by presenting the objectives for the unit. One can then stimulate recall of prior learning by a narrative in which the narrator says "Just think of the ability to modify older technology for application to new uses. For example, sonar has improved to the point that the resolution is much more powerful and user-friendly. Google Earth has opened the door to new opportunities to do preliminary searches to find areas worthy of full-scale archaeological expeditions." Having shared this with the student, it is time present the material to be learned. This could be done is relatively short interactive units. Student performance is elicited during this section with the provision of learner guidance. Also, in this section feedback should be provided in response to how the students respond to the interactive sections. A multiple-choice quiz could follow along with immediate feedback to his or her performance on the test. Retention and recall could be provided by closing with a moral to the instruction. "Archaeology has greatly benefitted from modification of older technology. We can see beneath the sea, beneath the obscuring jungle, beneath the surface of the earth itself. With this technology it is easier to find likely sites for excavation."

SUMMARY

A summary of the material presented in this book concludes this task. The information explosion has taken on a geometric progression that some feel that information will be doubling every 12 hours in the very near future. Keeping up with this and transforming information into knowledge assumes an ever-greater challenge. Neuroscientists are learning more and more about how the brain operates, which information is proving useful to educators. By using teaching techniques that encompass these idiosyncrasies of our brain, we can perhaps make learning more effective and more efficient. Instructional technology offers expanding opportunities in both online and offline settings to help achieve this goal of increased efficiency and effectiveness. Artificial intelligence offers a means to scan this information and make it more meaningful to the citizen of tomorrow.

REFERENCES

David, L. (2017). *Learning theories in plain English.* Retrieved from https://www.learning-theories.com/

Despopoulos, A., & Silbernagle, S. (1983). *Color atlas of physiology* (2nd ed.). New York, New York: Thieme, Inc.

Gagné, R. M. (1985). *The conditions of learning and theory of instruction* (4th ed.). New York, NY: Holt, Rinehart, and Winston.

Williams, C. W. (2003). *History of Jones County, Georgia 1807-1907: Memorial edition.* Fernandina Beach, FL: Wolfe Publishing.

Chapter 9
Education and the Future

ABSTRACT

How can educators prepare their students for the many changes brought about by the information explosion? It is taking longer for students to finish their undergraduate degrees; more women are successful with earning their degrees that are men. Occupations are disappearing and new ones appearing at increasing speed. Education is one approach, but a changed and more responsive education system will be necessary. Students must learn how to be lifelong learners and discover their interests and talents through aptitude testing followed by counseling. Though of great age, the lecture remains one of the best ways to transmit information and will likely last, but in a modified form. These changes will profoundly affect politics, economics, the environment, and other areas of our lives.

EDUCATION AND THE FUTURE

There are various consequences of the information explosion, many of them unanticipated. This proliferation of information and the knowledge made from it will affect all areas of society: occupations, political, economic, environmental. These changes will affect our very humanity. The question becomes—How do educators prepare the coming generations to deal with this change? Keeping up with the creation of new information will likely become more and more difficult. If it doubles every 12 hours, as some predict, humanity will soon be awash in information of all kinds. What shall, or can be done with it? How will that information be turned into knowledge? Teaching is difficult under

DOI: 10.4018/978-1-7998-1542-6.ch009

Figure 1.

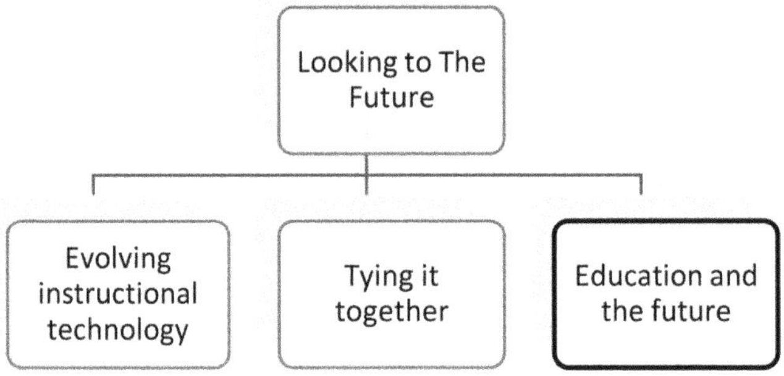

normal circumstances but imagine what it will be like to cover more and more material. Where will it end? Coupled with the general dissatisfaction with school performance on standardized tests, one can foresee in the near future a sea change in how education is viewed and conducted. When one of the authors was in school, practically everyone finished college in four years; he finished in little more than three years. Now, the norm has advanced to six years and more. According to "Undergraduate Retention and Graduation Rates" (2017), "About 59 percent of students who began seeking a bachelor's degree at a 4-year institution in fall 2009 completed that degree within 6 years; the graduation rate was higher for females than for males (62 percent vs. 56 percent)" (para. 1). There is also a lamentable failure to graduate that ranges from a high of 73% to a low of 27% (Fact Sheet: Focusing Higher Education on Student Success, 2015).

OCCUPATIONS

Occupational groups should be explored and examined. The Bureau of Labor Statistics *Occupational Outlook Handbook* lists 25 occupation groups representing 343 occupations. The occupations range from jobs requiring not even a high school diploma to professions and doctor's degrees. See Table 1 for a listing of these occupation groups. The occupations within these groups are expected to grow at an annual rate of seven percent for a 10-year period that was calculated to extend from 2016 to 2026 (*Occupational Outlook Handbook*, 2019).

It would be no stretch of the imagination to see a profession disappear before one who is preparing for it graduates from college or university. The

Table 1.

	Occupation Group	Occupations Within Occupation Group
1	Architecture & Engineering Occupations	25
2	Arts and Design Occupations	7
3	Building and Grounds Cleaning Occupations	3
4	Business and Financial Occupations	21
5	Community and Social Service Occupations	8
6	Computer and Information Technology	10
7	Construction and Extraction	19
8	Education, Training, and Library	13
9	Entertainment and Sports	8
10	Farming, Fishing, and Forestry	4
11	Food Preparation and Serving	6
12	Healthcare	45
13	Installation, Maintenance, and Repair	14
14	Legal	5
15	Life, Physical, and Social Science	29
16	Management	24
17	Math	3
18	Media and Communication	10
19	Military	25
20	Office and Administrative Support	13
21	Personal Care and Service	9
22	Production	15
23	Protective Service	6
24	Sales	10
25	Transportation and Material Moving	11
	Total Occupations	343

Compiled from Bureau of Labor Statistics on April 23, 2019. https://www.bls.gov/ooh/

father of one of the authors was a section foreman on the railroad. Then, in the early to mid-1950s, the railroads went into a decline. Competition from the trucking industry was too strong and ultimately won a significant share of the transportation market. At about the same time, diesel locomotives began to replace steam locomotives. The diesel engines were gentler on the tracks and, therefore, the profession of section foreman began to decline because the tracks required less maintenance.

The maritime industry declined in part due to being undercut by ships that were registered in other nations. The American unions were successful to the extent that they raised the pay of American seamen to the highest in the world. The United States could not compete with the lower shipping rates of other maritime nations. Consequently, the maritime industry of the United States began a steady decline.

Going back not too far in history, the pony express rider was a short-lived occupation, lasting only 19 months. It was replaced by the spread of the telegraph from coast to coast and the growth of the railroad. This is perhaps the shortest-lived occupation in history.

In years past, radio operators have served in the Navy, the Merchant Marine, and the CIA. The Central Intelligence Agency in 1974 was beginning to switch to satellite-based communications. Therefore, Morse code high frequency continuous wave and radioteletype were doomed to obsolescence as an occupation. This form of communication continuous wave (CW) transmission is no longer taught in the military and coast guard. There are no more stations monitoring 500khz for distress calls. The last commercial sea service Morse Code message was transmitted from a shore station in 1995. To hear a simulated distress call issued from the RMS Titanic in April of 1912 use these search terms: simulated titanic distress call (https://www.youtube.com/watch?v=snkwsU98QlQ). This simulation was transmitted using the spark-gap transmitters that were common in those early days. This even predates the SOS with which we are all familiar. Back then the distress call was CQD (meaning, calling all stations, distress). The speed of transmission in the simulation is about 20 to 25 wpm, which is rather fast. Later, it became a rule that distress messages could not be transmitted faster than 16 wpm. The only sector currently keeping Morse code alive is amateur radio (ham). Many occupations have become obsolete and are perhaps some on the verge of obsolescence.

Though some of the occupations were short-lived, they made a tremendous impact on the mythos of the United States. For example, consider the cowboy, this occupation extended from about 1865 to 1910 (45 years or thereabout). Even so, think of the profound impact this job had on our folklore. Consider the railroad locomotives, the paddlewheel riverboats, the majestic sailing vessels that plied the oceans of the world. Those occupations may have been of relatively short duration, but their impact was truly significant.

So, information explodes, knowledge derives from this information, occupations come into being and then owing to advancing technology fade into obscurity while some vanish into the mists of folklore. Peter Drucker (1998) alluded to this in the form of a question concerning the then new printing profession:

Printers were courted by kings, princes, the pope, and rich merchant cities and were showered with money and honors. ...Is there a lesson in this for today's information technologists, the CIOs in organizations, the software designers and developers, the devotees of Moore's Law?" (p. 9).

How then can educators train the young and not so young to enter new occupations?

EDUCATION

Education is likely to change to a radically different form from what it is today in 2019. Based on the previous section about occupations, we would be wise to spend time teaching young people how to learn so that they can become lifelong learners and have the capacity of keeping up with rapidly evolving technology and its impact on occupations. It would be wise to train or educate people so that they can apply their knowledge to new occupations. In the case of one of the authors, he discovered that many of the rules or habits governing radio communications network circuits apply to computer technology. Also, Morse code is digital in the sense that current flow (1) and non-current flow (0) is the same process for computers. Whereas the Morse code was a two-level (binary) code, radioteletype was a five-level code, computer languages is an eight-level or ASCII code. Often, new technology is so new and widely accepted at such a fast rate that insufficient time exists to create training programs to help new learners learn to use them.

It is likely that the lecture will remain a useful tool in the teacher's toolbox. Though much maligned in recent years, the traditional lecture remains a great method for imparting knowledge. Driscoll and Carliner (2005) observed that lectures are the most accurate way to present content, best to use for students for whom English is not their native tongue, the most efficient way to communicate content, as well as carrying other advantages. But, a lecture can be high tech and make great use of instructional technology.

Consider for a moment a "perfect" lecture. This perfect lecture could be about music of the Baroque Period from the early 1600s to the 1730 (Wildridge, 2019, March 11)—a time of tremendous advances in music, science, and other academic disciplines. The lecture could begin with some slides of Baroque Architecture and fashions. This introduction could be followed by an example of the music of that period—the great composers: Bach, Albinoni, Telemann, Handel, Vivaldi, Scarlatti, Rameau, Pachelbel, and others. The examples could be performances on period instruments (instruments that were popular in the Baroque period). One such excellent group is Il Giardino Armonico. You may wish to visit them on Youtube.com. The theorbo (archlute) is one instrument that was extremely popular back then but fell out of favor in modern orchestras. Even so, the sound is hauntingly beautiful, and its range is quite impressive. By the way, the great violin maker, Antonio Stradivarius, lived and built his violin family of instruments during this time.

A selection of these performances could be embedded within a PowerPoint slide show. During this presentation, the professor could provide a narrative to link these examples together. It could be a powerful experience that most students would likely remember for years to come. During a selection by Vivaldi, the professor could tell his or her class Vivaldi "did charity work for an orphanage for girls in which he trained the girls to play his compositions upon various instruments and had them perform in the cathedral. The talent of these young girls was quite remarkable in playing the various types of instruments in the violin family and the theorbo and the various kinds of wind instruments (recorder, oboe and so forth)." As the unit advances, selections of art and architecture could be featured in the visual and aural presentation. At Oglethorpe University in Atlanta, Georgia, the curriculum was strongly horizontally aligned. The music, literature, science, and other disciplines of the various great periods of Western civilization were studied in tandem. It was a marvelous and life-changing experience. Students at Oglethorpe were truly educated. This example could be followed in other disciplines and lectures.

The lecture began to play a reduced role in education in the latter part of the 20th century and the beginning of the 21st century. Other forms of pedagogy came to the forefront. These called upon students to become more active in their learning through collaboration. Evolving instructional technology found its place in this new age of teaching and learning. Access to the world wide web can play an increasingly important part in such classes. For example, consider a class on literature concerning the Middle English period, which included the 1400s—the time of Chaucer. Clearly, the English language has changed very much since those days. The class could be broken into two groups: the language of Chaucer, the language of today. What did Chaucer's Canterbury Tales sound like in the language of that day? This group could access the Internet and do a WebQuest of the spoken language of that period in history. The other group could meanwhile try to convert Chaucerian English into Modern English. They, too, could access the Internet and conduct a WebQuest. Once done, the two groups could combine and share the results of their labor. Then, the Chaucerian English group could conduct a class on how to speak Middle English, which could be a lot of fun and engaging to everyone in the class.

Technology can now make learning anywhere anytime a reality. Handheld digital devices could be used to gain access to the Internet and from the Internet the cloud which contains the authoring program and the learning material. Once done the student can take advantage of the short times during which he or she has little to do, such as during a break or while traveling on the bus or other forms of public transportation. Actually, the brain prefers this kind of instruction and can capitalize on this feature. Since the digital device (e.g. iPad) can serve as a "monitor" the learner can revel in the audio and the images. Even simple response mechanisms can be part of such a program. The biggest disadvantage of this form of learning is the lack of an adequate input device to permit the student to compose formal papers.

To get back to the issue of teaching, Sardana (n.d.) observes that

In the emerging scenario of digital environment, educators would be required to reorient their methodologies with a view to incorporating the digital based teaching aids and create among the students and also among themselves the curiosity levels to trigger a vision for looking at the things creatively so that students and teachers alike can visualize the gap between their present level of understanding and how digital aids can bridge such gaps (p. 8).

The need is to develop a functional level of digital literacy in students. "The educational curricula at different levels have to increasingly integrate the emerging digital culture blending all the mediums and the associated cultural perspectives through highly analytic and abstract literature of computational thinking enabled by computer software" (p. 9). Sardana (n.d.) additionally observes that "Their funding and the skills of teachers do not provide for necessary tools for the new literacy matching the digital world and culture" (p. 10). It is unknown about how successful this could become because not everyone has the aptitude or interest in learning such material, which sounds very much like statistics. It would be supposed that through constant exposure and much application would develop some degree of fluency in learners.

Digital literacy is only one part of a multipart problem. An even greater issue is preparing students to excel in new skill areas, many of which are not even currently known. One answer is to teach young people how to learn and how to obtain a wide view of the areas in which their aptitudes can guide them. Catering to one's aptitudes can create a strong foundation upon which to build many careers rather than one. McKay (2018), defines an aptitude as " referring to a natural talent or an ability an individual has acquired through life experience, study, or training. The word may also pertain to one's capacity to acquire a skill" (para. 2). This leads to making a distinction between an occupation and a job. Occupation is a much wider classification than a job because an occupation will likely include a rather large number of jobs. Aptitude is only one of several variables that one should consider in determining their career path(s). These other variables include one's personal interests, personality type, and work values. McKay (2018) pointed out that one could discover that he or she has an aptitude for more than one occupation. It is a very fluid, but a very important measure. It would be wise to administer aptitude tests to all students to narrow the focus of possibilities for future occupations so that they can realize early in their lives various occupations and jobs within occupations at which they might likely excel.

New recruits took the Armed Services Vocational Aptitude Battery (ASVAB) when they entered boot camp in the Navy in 1966. A recruit scored very high on an aptitude for Morse code. The Chief Petty Officer who counseled him said, "Son, looks like you would make a great radioman." The recruit responded, "Let's do it." The test was correct, he was an excellent radioman. Before that, when students entered the eighth grade, they were given an aptitude test. One of them scored 98 on music. The music faculty and counseling staff tried to recruit him for the band, but he resisted and took private music lessons. Aptitude tests can provide valuable insight into occupations in which one might excel and lay the groundwork for career changes in response to the effects of the information explosion.

POLITICS

Political structures will likely have to change to a more socialist democratic norm, depending on the wealth of the nation in which this is an issue and the will of its citizens. Even basic jobs will require sophisticated skills. The high school dropout will find it increasingly difficult to find employment. Even persons who have a high school diploma may prove only marginally more successful in finding work. A significant shift has occurred from manual labor to intellectual effort. About every aspect of life has had an encroachment of technology. For example, automobile mechanics must now be effective users of computing devices that control the operation of an automobile and that diagnoses problems. The same holds true for most of the trades and crafts that serve our society. No longer are ditches dug by hand, they are dug by machines who are operated by skilled craftsmen. Practically all strenuous manual labor has been replaced by machines the operation of which are governed by computers. Surveyors use GPS and more modern forms of transits to do their jobs accurately.

This move into technology could create societal and economic upheaval, which in turn might lead to political problems. The digital divide is rather sharp between have and have not nations and between the poor and the middle classes in the United States. Sardana (n.d.) provides a comment on this situation:

In the context of American Economy, the increasing inequalities is not a picture of healthy society. Such a level of economic inequality; not seen in the United States since the eve of the Great Depression, bespeaks a political economy in which the financial rewards are increasingly concentrated among a tiny elite whose risks are borne by an increasingly exposed and unprotected middle class. Income inequality in the United States is higher than in any advanced industrial democracy and by conventional measures comparable to that in countries such as Ghana, Nicargua [sic] and Turkmenistan. It breeds political polarization, mistrust, and resentment between the haves and have-nots and tend to distort the working of a democratic political system in which money increasingly confers political voice and power. It is generally presumed that economic forces alone are responsible for this astonishing concentration of wealth. Technological changes, particularly the information revolution, have transformed the economy, making workers more productive and placing a premium on intellectual, rather than manual labour (p.5).

Such conditions create a field ready for exploitation by politicians and demagogues. A discontent populace creates political instability and lays the groundwork for potential upheaval. In the current political climate, populism has resurfaced and shaken traditional political thought and action. A strong socialist slant is provided by various candidates for president. There is unrest on major university campuses where the more left-leaning students shout down and drive out those who present a conservative view. It is becoming increasingly hostile even toward our history with demands to remove statues and other memorials to the Confederacy and of some of our founding fathers. Congress, the presidency, and the supreme court seem to be unable to break the impasse. All seems to be driven by strong emotions. When strong emotions rule, there is little that reason, collaboration, and compromise can accomplish until cooler heads prevail. This situation bodes ill for the future.

How, then, can education help to promote and support a viable political system? From the experience of one of the authors, it seems that many Americans have a vague concept of how our republican form of government is supposed to run. There seems to be an idea abroad that we are a democracy, and we are, but our founders realized that it would be better to elect representatives to govern our nation; that a system of checks and balances be in place to prevent excess; and that majority rule can be contrary to the principles of democracy, thus leading to the concept of the tyranny the majority. Such a could be called mob rule. Stated differently, emphasis must be given to civics education. In higher education, these principles can also be retaught from time to time.

A disciplined and functioning democracy depends upon a strongly educated population. For education, this means teaching critical thinking skills; how to separate the wheat from the chaff; to cut through the bluster to the essence of a candidate's agenda. To consider the long-term consequences that can follow from decisions of state. To be able to deal with unintended consequences. To consider how to pay for mandated actions upheld by law. This leads one to wonder about what mechanisms could be used for these purposes. Formal debates can go far to achieve this end. One could provide for virtual trips to the legislature in action. Role-playing with students taking turns being the president, or a supreme court judge could provide vicarious experiences in decision making.

A high school curriculum based on *America, The Owner's Manual* (Graham, 2018) would be equally useful in higher education. According to Graham (2018), this curriculum in active citizenship rests upon five key principles:

- Help students recognize challenges or opportunities in their school, community, state, or nation that can be addressed through effective citizenship;
- Instruct students on the competencies required for civic success (i.e., the skills of effective citizenship);

- Provide students with a foundational knowledge of democratic institutions and processes while teaching citizenship skills (e.g., exploring federalism to identify which level of government can resolve the challenge a student has selected);
- Instill in students the dispositions of democratic citizenship, such as respect for fellow citizens of different races, religions, classes, and sexualities, and tolerance for different political viewpoints; and
- Encourage students to utilize their newly learned skills, knowledge, and values to address the challenge or opportunity they have identified (p. 7).

These principles suggest a constructivist approach to teaching the subject. Acting upon these principles implies applied learning, which is very powerful. This is also a very good example of how the education of our youth could be approached. One could begin by teaching principles, then ask his or her students to apply those principles. When one learns principles in addition to solid content, one tends to be able to apply them to new jobs while remaining within the same occupation group or even change to another occupation group. This helps to emphasize the power in knowing one's aptitudes. It creates a certain level of confidence that engenders success in excelling at new jobs that come into being as technology advances. However, the advantage lies in the power of intellectual effort rather than in manual labor.

ECONOMICS

Closely allied with politics is economics, and economics will lie at the foundation of any society that participates in the global market. Will there be enough jobs to provide economic security to the general population? Or, better stated, will the population be sufficiently educated to create general wellbeing? This, then, leads us to the realm of education, which is closely allied to both politics and economics. This also brings up the realm of gender differences. While IQ scores are essentially the same for women and men, women have a statically significant higher emotional IQ than do men, and furthermore "Emotional intelligence is responsible for 58% of performance in all types of jobs, and 90% of top performers are high in EQ" (Bradberry, 2016, para. 4).

Gone are the days when young men could find employment rather easily, though it was generally manual labor. In the 19th century and before most families were engaged in farming. Advancing technology and agricultural knowledge have drastically reduced the number of small farms. Now, ability with computers and the use of software are vital employment skills, even for farmers. Without a change in attitude toward learning and education, the welfare population would likely increase, which could bankrupt our economy. Another issue is the growing number of criminals in our society and the drain their upkeep takes from the economy. How can teachers and professors help to turn this situation around? There is no easy answer and no single solution because these problems are exacerbated by negative motivation or lack of motivation. These problems begin early in the lives of young people—in their infancy. Poor parenting and negative experiences in school have a strong influence on their development and potential economic success.

One step a professor in higher education could take is to require that a budget accompany each proposal project developed as assignments. One of the authors did that in a course on A Video Producer. One assignment was to convert a short story by Nathaniel Hawthorne, *The Hollow of Three Hills*, into a screenplay accompanied by a scene breakdown, locations, a production schedule, a talent list, and a budget. All these elements created a production book for the project. The short story was only 1,766 words in length, which made it a viable project for a single course. Furthermore, there were no copyright issues as the story was written in 1830 and the copyrights had expired. This proved to be an interesting assignment because it made the students consider all the elements that went into staging a production. Even short productions are complicated and difficult to execute. It raised their awareness of the many issues surrounding the process of creating a successful production of a dramatic video.

Much social upheaval in history was the result of economic imbalances among the population. It is easily summed up in the aphorism that the rich get richer and the poor get poorer. This creates a seemingly insoluble problem. Capitalism has proved to be extraordinarily successful but can create three classes: the poor, middle class, and rich. On the other hand, socialism and communism have failed everywhere it was tried; never once have these systems succeeded. It produced a system in which the great majority were equally impoverished. Educators in higher education could provide instruction and activities to delve into this problem so that students could get a first-hand idea of the workings of these economic systems.

ENVIRONMENT

Environmental concerns will assume greater importance in the future, particularly with the issue of global warming. That climate is changing is generally without doubt; the question is whether it is manmade or a natural cyclic progression of things or a combination of these. Higher education can help their students to come to terms with it and seek ways to create a steady climate. Currently, there is so much emotion surrounding the issue that reason has little opportunity to grapple the problem. Climate change is not a new phenomenon. In relatively modern times, the medieval warm period began 900 AD and extended until about 1300 AD (Rafferty, n.d.). This was followed by little ice age that featured two cooling episodes with slight warming between them (Rafferty & Stephen, n.d.). These began in about 1650 and the other in about 1760. There is further evidence to identify other periods of warming and cooling in prehistoric times. So, global warming is nothing new. In fact, this warming period may well be followed by another little ice age. Teachers and professors should urge caution and the use of reason when discussing these issues. It is an excellent opportunity to teach critical thinking skills.

Another issue is the increase in environmental pollution. Were the earth's environment compared to that of an aquarium, the waters are becoming increasingly fouled at a rate that the system cannot keep up with it and keep it clean. It seems that some kinds of human garbage are such that it is well-nigh indestructible, such as plastic and Styrofoam. Unless something is done to counteract this tendency to pollute the planet, it is not inconceivable that the entire earth will become one large landfill. Teachers and professors can help raise awareness of this issue and encourage their students to find ways to recycle our trash to keep the earth beautiful and fruitful.

Deforestation is gaining momentum with vast tracks of jungle being burned to make way for short term land use for farming. This is short term because that land has shallow topsoil and its nutrients are rapidly depleted by poor farming practices. The dust bowl in the United States is but one example of the results of over-farming without letting the land replenish itself (Klein, 20219). It is an oft-told tale of short-term benefits at the expense of long-term disaster. This situation lends itself to rational thought and education of youth to take steps to reverse this trend.

The earth's atmosphere is in part generated by a careful blend of sentient and non-sentient life. The plants and ocean algae breath in carbon dioxide and breath out oxygen. Animal life operates on the opposite principle; they breathe out carbon dioxide and breathe in oxygen. It is a symbiotic relationship. Yet, the world population is growing at astronomical rates and plant life is diminishing at the same time. There will eventually come a time of diminishing returns in which animal life, including human life, will become increasingly deprived of oxygen, which is a vital ingredient of our atmosphere. Awareness is part of the answer to turn this around.

Unbridled population growth is also a threat to human survival. In the 1600s, the worldwide human population was estimated to be 500 million. Four hundred years later, in the year 2000, worldwide population was estimated at approximately 6 billion and is estimated to become 9.8 billion in 2050. Estimates for 2019 are 7.346 billion people (*World Population*, May 4, 2019). Where are all these people coming from? The majority are coming from developing nations and those not as industrialized as the top economic powers. It would seem to be related to childbearing, prosperity and poverty. For example, According to *World Population* (May 4, 2019),

A few scientists even believe that populations will decrease. Some believe that gradual increases in living standards will result in similar patterns to those in Western Europe, where birth rates are declining rapidly. Others believe that the current world population is unsustainable and predict that humanity will simply not be able to produce enough food and oil to feed itself and sustain our industrial economy (para. 15).

The first prediction is preferable to the second; the second heralds an unthinkable alternative.

Birth rates are declining in many of the advanced nations. Nargund (2009) noted that

Fertility rates tend to be higher in poorly resourced countries but due to high maternal and perinatal mortality, there is a reduction in birth rates. In developing countries children are needed as a labour force and to provide care for their parents in old age. In these countries, fertility rates are higher due to the lack of access to contraceptives and generally lower levels of female education. The social structure, religious beliefs, economic prosperity and urbanization within each country are likely to affect birth rates as well as abortion rates. Developed countries tend to have a lower fertility rate due to lifestyle choices associated with economic affluence where mortality rates are low, birth control is easily accessible and children often can become an economic drain caused by housing, education cost and other cost involved in bringing up children. Higher education and professional careers often mean that women have children later in life. This can result in a demographic economic paradox (para. 1).

Economics does play a powerful role in population growth. Overall there seems to be a tendency in the more advanced nations to reduce childbearing for several reasons, one of which is economic. In developing nations, birth rates, though higher than in industrialized nations, are mitigated owing to various factors including infant and childhood mortality. Overall, the world population is growing with no end in sight, but there does seem to be a tendency toward stasis or a modest decline.

SUMMARY

The role of educators in this look into the future seems bright yet challenging. Most, if not all, global conditions can be viewed either positively or negatively. On the positive side, instructional technology can make learning more effective and efficient, but education is not solely able to turn around these problems. Also, it takes time for one generation to move from school to roles of leadership and participation to make the world a better place. The very nature of education must be rethought and redesigned to cope with the changes being created by the information explosion.

Chapter 10 contains examples demonstrated in four disciplines: history, science, literature, and archaeology.

REFERENCES

Bradberry, T. (2016). *Why women are smarter than men.* Retrieved from https://www.forbes.com/sites/travisbradberry/2016/06/21/why-women-are-smarter-than-men/#a1349c417e6e

Driscoll, M., & Carliner, S. (2005). *Advanced web-based training strategies: Unlocking instructionally sound online learning*. San Francisco, CA: Pfeiffer.

Drucker, P. F. (1998). *The next information revolution.* Retrieved from http://www.s-jtech.com/Peter%20Drucker%20-%20the%20Next%20Information%20Revolution.pdf

Fact sheet: Focusing higher education on student success. (2015). Retrieved from https://www.ed.gov/news/press-releases/fact-sheet-focusing-higher-education-student-success

Graham, B. (2018, Summer). Teaching civic engagement. *American Educator*, *42*(2). Retrieved from http://eds.a.ebscohost.com.contentproxy.phoenix.edu/eds/pdfviewer/pdfviewer?vid=1&sid=a6d86dac-a26d-4633-9035-081c06ec7a1f%40sessionmgr4009

Klein, C. (2019, March 21). *10 Things you may not know about the dust bowl*. Retrieved from https://www.history.com/news/10-things-you-may-not-know-about-the-dust-bowl

McKay, D. R. (2018). *Knowing your aptitude can help you choose a career*. Retrieved from https://www.thebalancecareers.com/what-is-aptitude-526175

Nargund, G. (2009). *Declining birth rate in developed countries: A radical policy re-think is required*. Retrieved from https://www.ncbi.nlm.nih.gov/pmc/articles/PMC4255510/

Occupational outlook handbook. (2019). Retrieved from https://www.bls.gov/ooh/architecture-and-engineering/home.htm

Rafferty, J. P. (n.d.). Medieval warm period. In *Encyclopaedia Britannica*. Retrieved from https://www.britannica.com/science/medieval-warm-period

Rafferty, J. P., & Stephen, T. J. (n.d.). The Little Ice Age. In *Encyclopaedia Britannica*. Retrieved from https://www.britannica.com/science/Little-Ice-Age

Sardana, M. M. K. (n.d.). *Information explosion, challenges and opportunities*. Retrieved from http://isid.org.in/pdf/DN1209.pdf

Undergraduate retention and graduation rates. (2017). Retrieved from https://nces.ed.gov/programs/coe/pdf/Indicator_CTR/coe_ctr_2017_05.pdf

Wildridge, J. (2019, March 11). *Brief history of classical music periods*. Retrieved from https://www.cmuse.org/brief-history-of-classical-music-periods/

World population. (2019). Retrieved from http://worldpopulationreview.com/continents/world-population/

Section 4
Examples

In the final chapter in the book a series of examples are presented: history, science, literature, and archaeology. Each example begins with an overview of the subject to be covered. The overview is divided into topics. Each topic is then covered. Gagne's nine instructional events is common to all overviews and topics. This is because the nine instructional events fit comfortably into all learning theories. Therefore, each example and the topics within them can rest on any of a number of learning theories. Example 1 concerns history in which the War Between the States from a southern perspective is presented in an overview and three topics. Example 2 falls within science in which action potentials is the subject. This consists of an overview and four topics. Example 3 concerns literature. It is covered in one overview and two topics. Example 4 concerns archaeology. The subject is technology applied to archaeology. It is covered with one overview and three topics.

Figure 1.

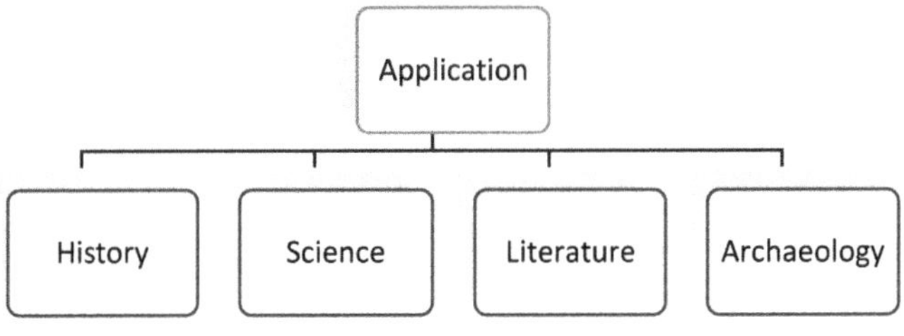

Chapter 10
Examples With Lesson Plans

ABSTRACT

The purpose of this final chapter is to provide examples of the application of the conceptual framework. This chapter contains lesson plans for four disciplines: history, science, literature, and archaeology. The four disciplines were chosen to represent science (action potentials and archaeology) and liberal arts (history and literature), all four of which are likely to be found in the curriculum of all universities. Each discipline has an overview element and plans for each of the topics within the units. Instructional technology is used in all the units of each of the disciplines. The methods used to impart the material can be any that the teacher chooses; however, most would work well with a constructivist approach. The nine instructional events developed by Dr. Robert Gagné can be used for all the units.

THE WAR BETWEEN THE STATES: A SOUTHERN PERSPECTIVE

This example will cover what the war felt like to a Southerner during the War Between the States. We shall follow a pattern for each of these examples.

Goal: To help students have a deeper understanding of how the people of the South felt about the War Between the States

Objectives:

1. Given the views expressed by Ms. Carolyn White Williams about the causes of the war use your critical thinking skills to examine their validity

DOI: 10.4018/978-1-7998-1542-6.ch010

Figure 1.

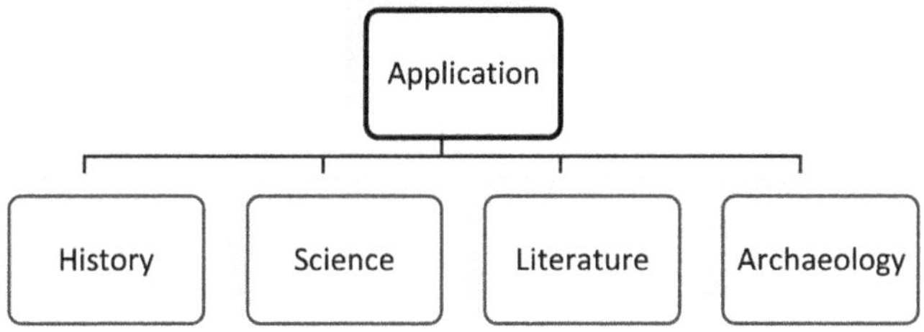

Figure 2.

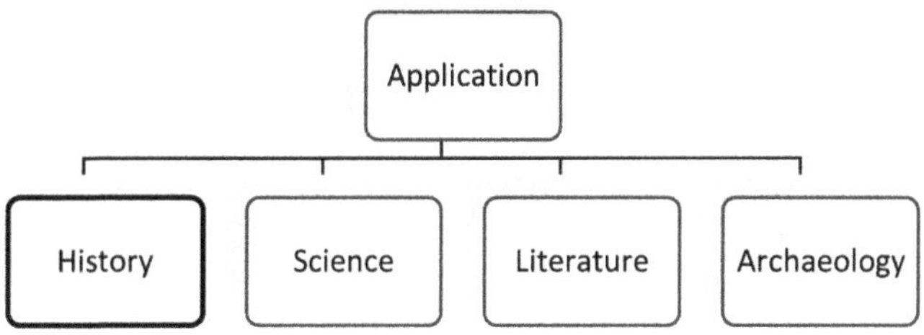

using a web quest to gather additional information and express your opinion in support of or contrary to this view in an essay of between 1000 and 1450 words.

2. Given the songs of the War Between the States era performed by Tom Roush, you will analyze the lyrics and state the three most common themes reflected in them with acceptable accuracy.
3. Given the readings about Sherman's march to the sea, you will present the event as viewed through the eyes of Georgians in the path of that march with adequate accuracy,
4. Given the websites describing the rebel yell, you will describe how the opposing troops may have reacted to it with satisfactory accuracy.
5. Given these materials, you will write an essay between 1,000 and 1,400 words about how they viewed the War Between the States, and why they felt that way.

Learner characteristics:

- Traditional college juniors aged between 20 and 25 years of age representing African-American, Hispanic, and Caucasian races and ethnicity.
- Learning theory: Constructivist
- Instructional design model: Gagne's nine instructional events (Gagné, 1985).
- Resources: computers, access to the Internet, handouts

Websites:

- Tom Roush *Battle Cry of Freedom* https://www.youtube.com/watch?v=NyWe2ILErVk
- *Listen to the Mockingbird* https://www.youtube.com/watch?v=5liOUZFVnAg
- *Lorena* https://www.youtube.com/watch?v=7U4yAXM53mI
- *Dixie's Land* https://www.youtube.com/watch?v=eLrg_k0iqPU
- *Sweet Evalina* https://www.youtube.com/watch?v=FmowHhmPyPw
- *Lily Dale* https://www.youtube.com/watch?v=Nf9bNa9mmAw
- *Sweet Virginia Belle* https://www.youtube.com/watch?v=zBoYIcK8xT0
- Civilian Account of Sherman's March to the Sea: http://www.thomaslegion.net/civilian_diary_sherman_march_to_the_sea_civil_war_newspaper.html
- This Day in Georgia Civil War History: https://georgiainfo.galileo.usg.edu/thisday/cwhistory/12/02/letter-from-augusta-eyewitness-account-of-march-to-the-sea-destruction
- Sherman's march; Journal of an eye-witness. https://www.nytimes.com/1864/12/23/archives/shermans-march-journal-of-an-eyewitness.html
- Women during the Civil War: https://www.georgiaencyclopedia.org/articles/history-archaeology/women-during-civil-war
- South will never forget Sherman's 'March to the Sea': https://www.dailyherald.com/article/20141115/news/141118831/

- The Rebel Yell Lives, Pt 1: https://www.youtube.com/watch?v=dfHylwlq9Ow
- What the Rebel Yell Sounded Like: https://www.youtube.com/watch?v=7mGAesLYIF8

Books:

- Lowe, J. C. & Hodges, S. (Eds.). (1998). *Letters to Amanda: The Civil War Letters of Marion Hill Fitzpatrick, Army of North Virginia (Civil War Georgia).* Macon GA: Mercer University Press.
- Williams, C. W. (2003). History of Jones County, Georgia 1807-1907. Fernandina Beach, FL: Wolfe Publishing. [see excerpts]

Topics:

Their attitudes were products of the times in which these individuals lived. We would be wise to avoid judging them and their deeds by modern standards. I find it odd that so much attention is directed toward diversity and multi-culturalism, while we do not extend that same courtesy to people of other times, which were certainly diverse and multi-cultural.

- Topic 1: Popular songs of the Civil War.
- Topic 2: Sherman's march to the sea as seen by Georgians in the path of that march.
- Topic 3: The rebel yell and its impact on opposing troops and attacking troops.
- Topic 4: Combine your responses to topics 1, 2, and 3 into a thoughtful essay of between 1400 and 1750 words that realistically reflects the attitudes and views of the Southern people, particularly those of Georgia.

Figure 3. Nine instructional events divided into three categories

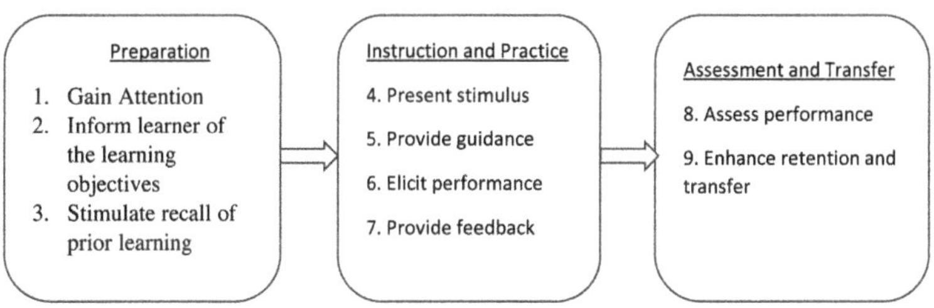

Table 1. Topic 1: nine instructional events by Gagne (1985, pp, 246-255)

The War Between the States: A Southern Perspective **Topic/lesson one: Causes of the War** **Using the views expressed by Ms. Carolyn White Williams about the causes of the war use your critical thinking skills to examine their validity. Conduct a WebQuest to gather information and express your opinion in support of or contrary to this view in an essay of between 1000 and 1450 words.**	
Preparation	
1. Gain attention	Ask a question: How would you feel if your country and home place were invaded by an enemy?
2. Inform about objectives	1. Research on the Internet to confirm or deny the views of Ms. Williams about the causes of the war/ 2. Analyze the lyrics of popular music of the time. 3. Describe your feelings about Sherman's March to the Sea. 4. Imagine the psychological impact the Rebel Yell had on the opposing forces. 5. Demonstrate empathy for the Southern view
3. Recall of prior knowledge	Have you ever felt bullied? Disrespected? Maligned? Falsely accused? What were your feelings? How did you respond?
Instruction & Practice	
4. Present material	Break into three groups. Group one analyzes the music to determine the top three themes. Group two presents the Georgians who were in the path response to Sherman's March to the Sea. Group three describes the impact the Rebel Yell had on the opposing forces.
5. Provide Guidance	Walk among the groups to monitor their progress and their ideas.
6. Elicit performance	Have each group present their findings to the class at large.
7. Provide feedback	Provide feedback about their conclusions, their work as a team, and their presentation
Assignment & Transfer	
8. Assess performance	Assign group grades in conjunction with peer grades
9. Enhance retention & transfer	Recap the lesson with a summary that includes a moral to the tale, which is the war could have been avoided and slavery abolished as in England under the urging of William Wilberforce. The agitation by the abolitionists was to a certain degree responsible for the conflagration that cost approximately 750,000 casualties (consisting of soldiers on both sides), yet these agitators are honored today though their hands are bloody from what they instigated. Seven hundred and fifty thousand lives lost, more than the combined total casualties of World War I, World War II, Korea, and Vietnam. Use this as a cautionary tale to think about those who are honored by society to see whether they are worthy of such honor and question what you have been led to believe.

A presentation of these three lessons about the Southern Perspective of the War Between the States using the nine instructional events devised by Gagné as depicted in Figure 3.

There were fanatics in the North who were unwilling to work out a plan to gradually free the slave without bringing ruin on the South. The fire-eaters preached hatred of the Southern people and slavery, they encouraged the millions of slaves to rise against their masters and burn and murder at will. With one-third of the South slaves, a prospect of uprisings brought terror to every Southern home. This and other acts of an unfriendly section, led the

Table 2. Topic 2: nine instructional events by Gagne (1985, pp. 246-255)

The War Between the States: A Southern Perspective Topic/Lesson two: What does the popular music of that day tell us about how the people felt about the war? The popular music of that time in history tells us how many of the common people on both sides felt about the war. Analyze the lyrics of three of these songs to determine what they are saying.	
Preparation	
1. Gain attention	Play the song Lorena and ask the class: What does this music say to them? After capturing their attention, announce the topic and purpose of the lesson.
2. Inform about objectives	1. Categorize the themes of the songs listed under resources. You may wish to use NVivo or a similar program to conduct the analysis. 2. Determine the top three themes. 3. Are these themes limited to that great struggle, or do they apply to all wars?
3. Recall of prior knowledge	Though most of you are too young to have experienced the war protests against our conflict in South Vietnam, you may wish to listen to some of the songs of that era.
Instruction & Practice	
4. Present material	Break into three groups. Group one analyzes the lyrics of Listen to the Mockingbird. Group two analyzes the lyrics of Sweet Evalina. Group three analyzes Lily Dale.
5. Provide Guidance	Walk among the groups to monitor their progress and their ideas.
6. Elicit performance	Have each group present their findings to the class at large.
7. Provide feedback	Comment on the presentations and ask questions of the class at large.
Assignment & Transfer	
8. Assess performance	Assign group grades in conjunction with peer grades
9. Enhance retention & transfer	Recap the lesson with a summary that includes a moral to the tale, which is that many music critics look down upon the music of the 19th century as being overly sentimental, but one wonders if this is the case. Death was more common in those days than now owing to diseases such as tuberculosis (consumption), poor maternity care produced many deaths of young women and their babies. So, I wonder if that music is really overly sentimental. Music is supposed to affect the emotions and the sentiments.

Southerners to leave the Union and to form their own government, one which would give protection to their families and homes. Propaganda helped to bring about the Civil War as much as anything else. Yes, the Southerners were haughty and proud and little disposed to consider the institution of slavery a pertinent topic to be discussed only among themselves. It was a question that might have with calm deliberation, been settled amicably by statesmen, but the agitation was begun and carried too far by rabid preachers and agitators and when an attempt was made in the eleventh hour to avert the pending catastrophe, too much passion had been aroused on both sides for a settlement to be possible. The war was a clash between divergent civilizations and rival economies, Northern powers seeking to exploit the South as a colony, which they did for ten years after the South conceded defeat (Williams, p. 101).

Table 3. Topic 3: nine instructional events by Gagne (1985, pp. 246-255)

The War Between the States: A Southern Perspective **Topic/lesson three: The Rebel Yell** **No one knows for sure the origin of the Rebel Yell. Some maintain that it was a hunting cry to rally the hounds; others maintain that it was descended from the Celtic war cry. You might also recognize elements of the war cry of Native Americans. It did, however, serve a powerful psychological purpose. There are accounts of different Confederate companies becoming engaged in a contest of such yelling.**	
Preparation	
1. Gain attention	Play the Rebel Yell from the internet without the preceding or the following narrative.
2. Inform about objectives	1. Read accounts of the effects of the yell from Union descriptions of it. 2. Conduct a WebQuest on the psychological power of such war cries. I believe that even Julius Caesar described such yelling from the Celtic and Germanic tribes in Europe. 3. Imagine the impact of this yelling on the Confederate soldiers themselves. They are marching toward the Union defenses, minnie balls and grapeshot was whizzing past them, the cannon and rifle fire was blasting away.
3. Recall of prior knowledge	Do you recall newscasts of various demonstrations in which the demonstrators were yelling and chanting? Or, cheering on your team during a football game. Perhaps this is but a version of the impact of and purpose of the Rebel Yell.
Instruction & Practice	
4. Present material	Divide the class into three groups. One to conduct a WebQuest to find descriptions of the yell by Union soldiers. The second group will find information on the Internet about Julius Caesar's descriptions of the Celtic warriors. The third group will find information about how the yell impacted friend and foe during the battles of the War Between the States.
5. Provide Guidance	Walk among the groups to monitor their progress and their ideas.
6. Elicit performance	Have each group present their findings to the class at large.
7. Provide feedback	Comment on the presentations and ask questions of the class at large.
Assignment & Transfer	
8. Assess performance 9.	Assign group grades in conjunction with peer grades Recap the lesson with a summary that includes a moral to the tale, which is that these three classes saw the invasion as an event that turned their lives upside down, but for different reasons. Even the slaves were unable to entirely endorse the event.

Excerpts for the history discipline:
Williams, C. W. (2003). History of Jones County, Georgia 1807-1907. Fernandina Beach, FL: Wolfe Publishing.
Carolyn White Williams

If you could have asked a Confederate soldier why the South seceded, he would probably have given the following reasons ("Facts the Historians Leave Out" by John S. Tilly): 1. Our states went with the Union with the understanding that they had the right to withdraw. When membership proved unhappy, we exercised that right. 2. We were sick and tired of being gypped by harsh tariff laws which enriched the North at our expense. 3. We were fed up with insane abuse from a group of South-hating fanatics. 4. Northerners had inspired murderous slave uprisings; why should we sit by and wait for more? 5. The Republicans preaching hatred for the South, had elected a president, who as we had reason to know was not our friend. 6. We had bought our slaves from Northerners; it seemed hardly fair for the North to take them away from us without at least returning some of the money which we had paid for them. 7. With New England lording itself as superior to all other sections, why should we tolerate such snobbish airiness? 8. We had no idea of making war on the North. Lincoln's reinforcement at Sumter brought about the bombardment. All that we wished and planned for was to go our own way and be let alone. (Williams, pp. 104-105).

I recall hearing Shelby Foote stated, "The answer a Southerner would give you as to "why are you are fighting?" if you were a Northerner, he would say: "I'm fighting because you're down here." He was being invaded and he thought … to defend his home." https://huntthedevil.wordpress.com/2015/07/07/because-youre-here/

Note: William Wilberforce led the successful movement in England to abolish slavery in the British Empire in 1833 (The Abolition Project, 2009). It is highly likely that we could have done the same here in the United States without engaging in a bloody war in which about 750,000 young men died. The Northern fanatics and zealots have much blood on their hands.

Figure 4.

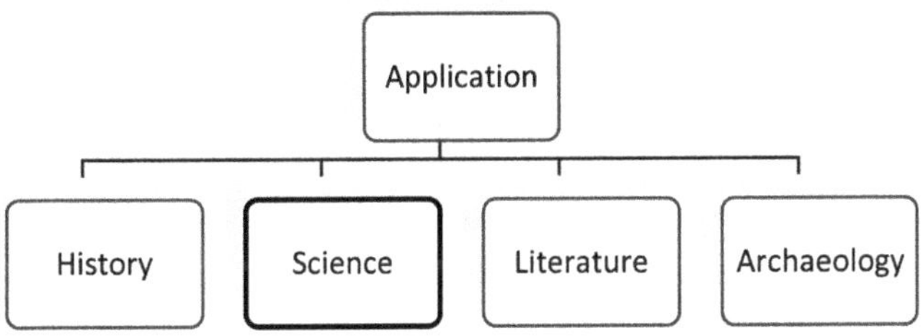

EXAMPLE 2

Science: Action Potentials

Action Potentials

This example will cover what generates and directs the path of the electrical impulses that govern the contracture of muscles, neurons, and endocrine cells.

Goal: To help students understand how life depends upon electrical impulses generated in cells and transmitted via nerves.

Objectives:

1. Given initial instruction and the results of a WebQuest, you will describe how electrical impulses are generated and propagated in a manner that is understandable.
2. Given initial instruction and viewing the resources you will describe how the electrical gradient inside the cell and the electrical gradient outside the cell seek to become equalized and thereby create a voltage spike with reasonable accuracy.
3. Given initial instruction and viewing the resources you will draw a graph of the Action Potential Cycle showing the resting potential, depolarization, repolarization, hyperpolarization, and resting membrane potential with complete accuracy
4. Given initial instruction and viewing the resources you will describe the process of electrical conduction along an axon to a synapse to end at a muscle cell to cause it to contract with clarity and precision.

Learner characteristics:

- Traditional college juniors representing African-American, Hispanic, and Caucasian races and ethnicity.
- Learning theory: Cognitivism
- Instructional design model: Gagne's nine instructional events (Gagné, 1985, pp, 246-255)
- Resources: Computers, access to the Internet, handouts

Websites:

- Calcium signaling in glial cells: https://video.search.yahoo.com/search/video;_ylt=AwrJ7Ju.O7VcP_IA3ONXNyoA;_ylu=X3oDMTE0dDl1NXNyBGNvbG8DYmYxBHB vcwMxBHZ0aWQDQjcw MTNfMQRz ZWMDcGl2cw--?p =calcium+signaling&fr2=piv-web&fr =yfp-t#id=28&vid =99bf8f9532f7672b150631f5f079bc82 &action=view
- High-magnification video of calcium signaling in astrocytes: https://video.search.yahoo.com/search/video; _ylt=AwrJ7Ju. O7VcP _IA3ONXNyoA; _ylu=X3oDMTE0dDl1NXN yBGNvbG8DYmYxBHB vcwMxBHZ0aWQDQ jcwMTNfMQR zZWMDcGl2cw --?p=calcium+ signaling&fr2= piv-web&fr=yfp -t#id=32&vid= cab5f817eb97204 e9698548f31025a6e &action=view
- Myocardial Action Potential: animation video: https://video.search.yahoo.com/search/video; _ylt=AwrC5pnLO7V cnSMAMSL7w8QF; _ylu=X3oDMTBncG dyMzQ0BHNlY wNzZWFy Y2gEdnRpZAM-; ylc=X1MDOTY3ODE zMDcEX3IDMgRhY 3RuA2NsawRiY2s DYnY2OWxtMWU2NzZmaS UyNmIlM0Q zJTI2cyUzRGF oBGNzcmNwdmlkA 3NIdHFSVEV 3TGpHX21UV 3dYR09aO GdSck9Ea 3VNUUFBQUFCb m9reHEEZnID eWZwLXQEZnIyA 3NhLW dwBGdwcmlkA0Z3 MHJwc1hpUlhTelF vWXIxTDBS c0EEbXRlc 3RpZANudW xsBG5fcn NsdAM2MAR uX3N1 Z2cDMTAEb 3JpZ2luA3 ZpZGVvLnNlYXJ jaC55YWhvby5jb 20EcG9zAzME cHFzdHIDYW N0aW9uIHBvdGVud GlhbARwcXN0cmw DMTYEcXN0cmw DMjYEcXV lcnkDYWN0aW9 uIHBvdGVudGlhb CBhbmltYXRpb 24EdF9zdG1w AzE1NTU zODE0O DcEdnR lc3RpZANu dWxs?gprid= Fw0rpsXiRXSz QoYr1L0RsA&pvid= sHtqRTEwLjG_mTWwXGOZ 8gRrODku MQAAAA Bnokxq&p=action+ potential+animation &ei=UTF- 8&fr2=p% 3As%2Cv% 3Av%2Cm% 3Asa&fr=yfp- t#id= 7&vid=07a1a1206e 932a8f40643913 ff6e9276&action=view
- Depolarization and Repolarization: https://video.search.yahoo.com/search/video; ylt=AwrC5pnLO7V cnSMAMSL7w8QF; _ ylu=X3oDMTB ncGdyMz Q0BHNlY wNzZWFyY2 gEdnRpZAM-; _ylc=X1MDOTY 3ODEzMD cEX3IDMg RhY3Ru A2NsawRi Y2sDYn Y2OWxtMWU 2NzZmaSUy NmIlM0Qz JTI2cyUzRGF oBGNzcm NwdmlkA 3NIdH FSVEV 3TGpHX21 UV3dYR09a OGdSck9Ea 3VNUUFBQUF Cbm9reHEEZ nIDeWZ wLXQEZnIy A3NhLWdwB GdwcmlkA0 Z3MHJwc1hpUlh TelFvWXIx TDBSc0EEbXRlc3R pZANud WxsBG5fcn NsdAM2MAR uX3N1Z2c

DMTAEb3 JpZ2luA3Zp ZGVvLnNlY XJjaC55 YWhvby5jb2 0EcG9zAzME cHFzdHIDYWN0a W9uIHBvdGV udGlhbARwc XN0 cmwDMTYE cXN0cmwDMjYE cXVlcnkDYWN0 aW9uIHBvdGV udGlhbCBhbmlt YXRpb24EdF 9zdG1w AzE1NTUz ODE0ODc EdnRlc3Rp ZANudWxs? gprid=Fw0rpsXiRXSzQ oYr1L0RsA &pvid=sHtqRTE wLjG_mTWw XGOZ8gRrOD kuMQAAAAB nokxq&p= action+ potential+ animation&ei=UTF- 8&fr2=p%3 As%2Cv%3 Av%2Cm%3 Asa&fr=yfp-t#id= 46&vid=cf07ad 7d40ccf5584 c2332eb6fc 18768&action=view

- Formation of Action Potentials: https://video.search.yahoo.com/ search/video;_ ylt=AwrC5pnLO7V cnSMAMSL7w8QF; _ ylu=X3oDMT BncGdyMzQ0BHNl YwNzZWFyY2 gEdnRpZAM-; _ylc=X1MDOTY3 ODEzMDcEX3 IDMgRhY3 RuA2NsawRiY2 sDYnY2OW xtMWU2 NzZmaSUy NmIlM0Qz JTI2cyUzRGF oBGNzcmNwdmlkA3NIdHFSVEV3TGpHX21UV3dYR09aOGdSck 9Ea3VNUUFB QUFCbm9re HEEZnID eWZwL XQEZnIy A3NhLWdw BGdwcmlk A0Z3MHJ wc1hpUlhTel FvWXIxTD BSc0EEbXR lc3RpZANud WxsBG5fcnNsd AM2MARuX3N1Z2 cDMTAEb 3JpZ2luA3ZpZ GVvLnNlYXJ jaC55YWhvby 5jb20EcG9 zAzMEcHF zdHIDYWN0 aW9uIHBvd GVudGlhbARwc XN0cmwDMTY EcXN0cmwDMjYEcX VlcnkDYWN0aW9uI HBvdGVudGlhb CBhbmltYXRpb 24EdF9zdG1 wAzE1NTUz ODE0ODcEdnRlc 3RpZANud Wxs?gprid= Fw0rpsXiRXSz QoYr1L0RsA&pvid= sHtqRTEwLjG_ mTWwXGOZ8 gRrODkuMQAAAA Bnokxq&p=action+ potential+animation &ei=UTF-8&fr2= p%3As%2Cv% 3Av%2Cm% 3Asa&fr=yfp- t#id=2&vid= 089c50f4efa 6914556464f05 dacc9548&action=view

Topics:

1. How action potentials (electrical impulses) are generated and sustained.
2. How the exterior and the interior of the cell membrane become equalized as is the case when there is no communication between and among the cells.
3. A graph of the action potentials showing the resting potential, depolarization repolarization, hyperpolarization, and resting membrane potential

Table 4. An overview: nine instructional events by Gagne (1985, pp. 246-255)

Action Potentials: An Overview	
Preparation	
1. Gain attention	Show the scene from *Frankenstein* in which lightening is attracted and infused into the carcass to bring the monster to life. When this scene ends, provide some general remarks to introduce the topic of instruction. One could say "Pretty intense is it not? And, not entirely true, but our bodies do work because of electrical impulses. Just how does this happen? Thus, we enter the world of action potentials."
2. Inform about objectives	1. Given initial instruction and the results of a WebQuest, you will describe how electrical impulses are generated and propagated in a manner that is understandable. 2. Given initial instruction and viewing the resources you will describe how the electrical gradient inside the cell and the electrical gradient outside the cell seek to become equalized and thereby create a voltage spike with reasonable accuracy. 3. Given initial instruction and viewing the resources you will draw a graph of the Action Potential Cycle showing the resting potential, depolarization repolarization, hyperpolarization, and resting membrane potential with complete accuracy 4. Given initial instruction and viewing the resources you will describe the process of electrical conduction along an axon to a synapse to end at a muscle cell with clarity and precision.
3. Recall of prior knowledge	Have you ever wondered how your digital devices are powered? The electricity that causes all your home and auto appliances to operate is also how your bodies are powered.
Instruction & Practice	
4. Present material	Let us begin with how these electrical charges are generated. Go to Formation of Action Potentials and view the animation. Once done, write a brief statement about how this occurs. Repeat with Depolarization and Repolarization. Repeat with myocardial action potential.
5. Provide Guidance	Call on various members of the class to read their statement. As these are read, correct errors as they appear. Repeat with Depolarization and Repolarization. Repeat with myocardial action potential.
6. Elicit performance	Break the class into two to four groups and have them find a suitable animation of the principles taught under item five Once done, each group should present their findings to the entire class.
7. Provide feedback	Provide feedback about their conclusions, their work as a team, and their presentation
Assignment & Transfer	
8. Assess performance	Assign group grades in conjunction with peer grades
9. Enhance retention & transfer	Reinforce what they have learned by showing them video of calcium signaling, which demonstrates these principles in action. End with a comment or moral of the story. "Our bodies are very busy places with all kinds of actions taking place without our conscious awareness. We have just seen how electricity powers our bodies. It is rather miraculous that this natural phenomenon animates our bodies and our minds."

Figure 5.

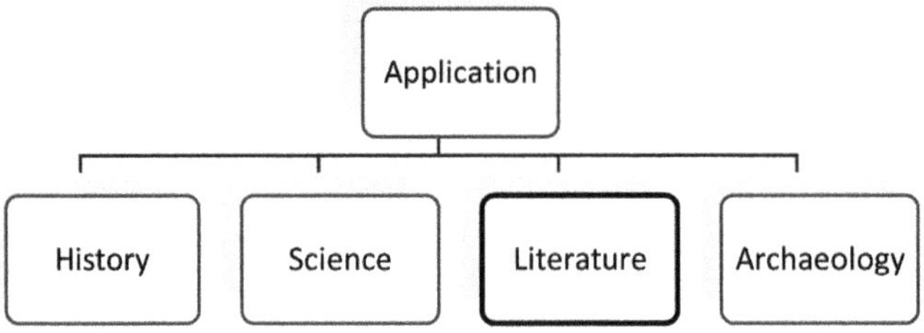

Table 5. Topic 1: nine instructional events by Gagne (1985, pp. 246-255)

Science: Action Potentials **Topic/lesson 1: The human body is powered by electrical signals/impulses.**	
Preparation	
1. Gain attention	Show calcium signaling in the cardiac cells. This kind of calcium signaling permits us to see the patterns of cell activity in the heart. In this instance, it is the heart of the zebra fish.
2. Inform about objectives	1. How are these electrical signals/impulses generated? 2. How are these impulses sustained?
3. Recall of prior knowledge	Just about every modern convenience is powered by electricity: your computers, cell phones, lights in the home and on the street that have freed humanity from the power of the darkness of the night.
Instruction & Practice	
4. Present material	The cognitivist approach is used with delivery by lecture and practice to apply the new knowledge.
5. Provide Guidance	As you explain and illustrate the subject, ask questions to which you will respond with either affirmation of the correctness of the response or provide corrective instruction in the event of a wrong answer.
6. Elicit performance	After delivering the information, ask students to explain it to the class.
7. Provide feedback	Comment on the presentations and ask questions of the class at large.
Assignment & Transfer	
8. Assess performance	Assign grades in conjunction with peer grades
9. Enhance retention & transfer	Recap the lesson with a summary that includes a moral to the tale, which is that electrical energy is easily generated by chemical actions.

4. How the action potential is generated along the length of the axon (nerve cell) to the synapse that connects to either another axon or to a muscle cell.

EXAMPLE 3

Literature

Literature: Folk Stories and Ballads as Literature

This example will cover the relationship of folk stories and folk ballads to literature.

Goal: To help students grasp the role of folk tales and ballads in entertaining the people and relate it to literature.

Objectives:

Table 6. Topic 2: nine instructional events by Gagne (1985, pp. 246-255)

Science: Action Potentials **Topic/lesson 2: How the voltage is generated** **The voltage in the cells is generated by permeability of the cell membrane that allows exchange of potassium and sodium ions that, in turn affect the polarity of the membrane.**	
Preparation	
1. Gain attention	Show an animation of the process by which an action potential is generated.
2. Inform about objectives	1. How are these electrical signals/impulses generated? 2. How are these impulses sustained?
3. Recall of prior knowledge	About every modern convenience is powered by electricity: your computers, cell phones, lights in the home and on the street that have freed humanity from the power of the darkness of the night.
Instruction & Practice	
4. Present material	Use the cognitivist approach with delivery by lecture and individual practice to apply the new knowledge.
5. Provide Guidance	As you explain and illustrate the subject, ask questions to which you will respond with either affirmation of the correctness of the response or provide corrective instruction in the event of a wrong answer.
6. Elicit performance	After delivering the information, ask students to explain it to the class.
7. Provide feedback	Comment on the presentations and ask questions of the class at large.
Assignment & Transfer	
8. Assess performance	Assign grades in conjunction with peer grades
9. Enhance retention & transfer	Recap the lesson with a summary that includes a moral to the tale, which is that electrical energy is easily generated by chemical actions.

Table 7. Topic 3: nine instructional events by Gagne (1985, pp. 246-255)

Science: Action Potentials Topic/lesson 3: Life Cycle of an Action Potential Graph the stages of the action potentials showing the resting potential, depolarization, repolarization, hyperpolarization, and resting membrane potential.	
Preparation	
1. Gain attention	Show an animated graph that depicts the cycle of an action potential.
2. Inform about objectives	1. What are the stages of an action potential cycle? 2. What stimulates the firing of an action potential?
3. Recall of prior knowledge	Just as an oscilloscope can depict the action of an oscillating current, so can action potentials be also graphed.
Instruction & Practice	
4. Present material	Use the cognitivist approach with delivery by lecture and individual practice to apply the new knowledge.
5. Provide Guidance	As you explain and illustrate the subject, ask questions to which you will respond with either affirmation of the correctness of the response or supply corrective instruction in the event of a wrong answer. End with students graphing the cycle of an action potential.
6. Elicit performance	After delivering the information, ask students to explain the graph to the class.
7. Provide feedback	Comment on the presentations and ask questions of the class at large.
Assignment & Transfer	
8. Assess performance	Assign grades in conjunction with peer grades
9. Enhance retention & transfer	Recap the lesson with a summary that includes a moral to the tale, which is that action potentials have a life cycle. Further, once the threshold is reached the additional magnitude of the pulse makes no difference in the creation of an action potential; therefore, the electrical impulse is primarily digital (no action potential equals zero; an action potential equals one).

1. Given the folk songs *Banks of the Ohio* and *Tom Dooley*, you will analyze the lyrics so that you can compare the two songs with credibility.
2. Given the songs listed in the resources, compare the subject matter of them with credibility.
3. Given the *Hollow of Three Hills* by Nathaniel Hawthorne, *Young Goodman Brown* (also by Hawthorne) and *Brer Rabbit and the Tar Baby* by Joel Chandler Harris describe how these stories reflect the genre of both folk tales and literature with credibility.

Learner characteristics:

Table 8. Topic 4: nine instructional events by Gagne (1985, pp. 246-255)

Science: Action Potentials **Topic/lesson 4: Mechanism of Flow** **How the action potential is generated along the length of the axon (nerve cell) to the synapse that connects to either another axon or to a muscle cell?**	
Preparation	
1. Gain attention	Show an animation of the progress of an action potential along an axon. When it reaches a synapse, a neurotransmitter carries the stimulus across the synapse at which time it continues its progress until it reaches a muscle cell and causes it to contract.
2. Inform about objectives	1. How is the action potential propagated along the length of an axon? 2. How does the synapse work?
3. Recall of prior knowledge	Just as an oscilloscope can depict the action of an oscillating current, so can action potentials be also graphed.
Instruction & Practice	
4. Present material	Use the cognitivist approach with delivery by lecture and individual practice to apply the new knowledge.
5. Provide Guidance	As you explain and illustrate the subject, ask questions to which you will respond with either affirmation of the correctness of the response or provide corrective instruction in the event of a wrong answer. End with students graphing the cycle of an action potential.
6. Elicit performance	After delivering the information, ask students to explain the graph to the class.
7. Provide feedback	Comment on the presentations and ask questions of the class at large.
Assignment & Transfer	
8. Assess performance	Assign grades in conjunction with peer grades
9. Enhance retention & transfer	Recap the lesson with a summary that includes a moral to the tale, which is action potentials flow along myelinated and non-myelinated nerve fibers. The progress is quite rapid and is measured in meters per second (m/s).

- Traditional college juniors representing African-American, Hispanic, and Caucasian races and ethnicity.
- Learning theory: Cognitivist
- Instructional design model: Gagne's nine instructional events
- Resources: computers, access to the Internet, handouts

Websites:

- *Young Goodman Brown*: http://andromeda.rutgers.edu/~jlynch/Texts/younggoodmanbrown.html

- *The Hollow of the Three Hills*: https://americanliterature.com/author/nathaniel-hawthorne/short-story/the-hollow-of-the-three-hills
- *Banks of the Ohio*: https://www.youtube.com/watch?v=5w8At8Aizx4
- *Tom Dooley*: https://www.youtube.com/watch?v=Bfb403ZQ-gU
- *Scarboro Fair*: https://www.youtube.com/watch?v=-BakWVXHSug and https://www.youtube.com/watch?v=x9_bluYa9Xc

Topics:

1. How are *Banks of the Ohio* and *Tom Dooley* alike and different?
2. How is the subject matter of the songs in the resources alike and different?
3. Describe how *Hollow of Three Hills* by Nathaniel Hawthorne, *Young Goodman Brown* (also by Hawthorne) and *Brer Rabbit and the Tar Baby* by Joel Chandler Harris reflect the genre of both folk tales and literature with credibility.

EXAMPLE 4

Archaeology

Archaeology: Technology

This example will cover the roles played by technology in archeological research.

Goal: To help students understand how archeologists use technology to further their discipline and science.

Objectives:

Figure 6.

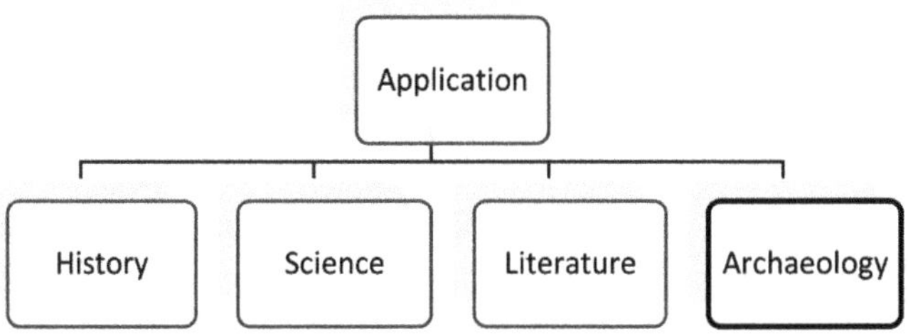

Table 9. Topic 1: nine instructional events by Gagne (1985, p. 246-255)

Literature: Folk Stories and Ballads as Literature Topic/lesson 1: How are Banks of the Ohio and Tom Dooley and other ballads alike and different? How is the subject matter of the songs in the resources alike and different?	
Preparation	
1. Gain attention	Begin: Play *Barbara Allen* and introduce the topic of folklore and literature. I like to think of folk stories as stories of everyday people that tells the events of an occurrence either seriously or with humor.
2. Inform about objectives	1. How are *Battle of New Orleans (The 8th of January)* and The *Battle of Antietam Creek* musically alike and different? 2. How is the content of the *Battle of New Orleans (The 8th of January)* and *The Battle of Antietam Creek* alike and different?
3. Recall of prior knowledge	Recall a news event that sticks in your mind. Think of it in terms of a story told to music.
Instruction & Practice	
4. Present material	Use the cognitivist approach with delivery by lecture and individual practice to apply the new knowledge. It would be both relevant and effective were there persons in the class who played a musical instrument and could sing a folk tale or folk song.
5. Provide Guidance	As you explain and illustrate the subject, ask questions to which you will respond with either affirmation of the correctness of the response or provide corrective instruction in the event of a wrong answer. End with students reciting the lyrics or even singing the lyrics of a song of their choice.
6. Elicit performance	After delivering the information, ask students to explain the words and describe the event in their own words.
7. Provide feedback	Comment on the presentations and ask questions of the class at large.
Assignment & Transfer	
8. Assess performance	Assign grades in conjunction with peer grades
9. Enhance retention & transfer	Recap the lesson with a summary that includes a moral to the tale, which is songs serve at least two purposes: 1) entertain and 2) inform. That they are set to music makes them easier to remember and to repeat. The power of music to help our memory is of great significance and proven to be effective.

1. Given the presentation on technology applied to archaeology, you will describe the uses of LIDAR, Google Earth, side scan sonar, and ground penetrating radar clearly and concisely.
2. Given Google Earth, you will select an area of the earth and search it for traces of ancient civilizations by finding one such example.
3. Given access to the Internet and a computer, you will conduct a WebQuest to identify an example of the uses of archaeology technology with success.

Learner characteristics:

Table 10. Topic 2: nine instructional events by Gagne (1985, p. 246-255)

Literature: Folk Stories and Ballads as Literature **Topic/lesson 2: Folk Tales with a Moral** **The Hollow of Three Hills by Nathaniel Hawthorne, Young Goodman Brown (also by Hawthorne) and Brer Rabbit and the Tar Baby by Joel Chandler Harris reflect the genre of both folk tales and literature with credibility**	
Preparation	
1. Gain attention	Begin: Play an audio recording of the *Hollow of Three Hills*. This is a very short story and could be read between 12 and 17 minutes.
2. Inform about objectives	1. How is this literary composition like a folk story? 2. Does this literary form help or hurt the story?
3. Recall of prior knowledge	Do any of you know any folk tales? I do. I know several of them. How does a folk take resemble a fairy tale? Is there a resemblance?
Instruction &Practice	
4. Present material	Use the cognitivist approach with delivery by lecture and individual practice to apply the new knowledge. Have the class silently read the *Tar Baby*. Ask: What is the moral of this tale? These kinds of stories tend to span different cultures in different parts of the world. Where did the story told by Joel Chandler Harris originate? It was in West Africa.
5. Provide Guidance	As you explain and illustrate the subject, ask questions to which you will respond with either affirmation of the correctness of the response or provide corrective instruction in the event of a wrong answer. End with a discussion about *The Legend of Sleepy Hollow*.
6. Elicit performance	After delivering the information, ask students to explain the words and describe the event in their own words.
7. Provide feedback	Comment on the presentations and ask questions of the class at large.
Assignment & Transfer	
8. Assess performance	Assign grades in conjunction with peer grades
9. Enhance retention & transfer	Recap the lesson with a summary that includes a moral to the tale, which is that these tales serve at least two purposes: 1) entertain and 2) inform. They are a form of literature that is so ancient that it originates before humanity was literate. One can easily imagine our ancient ancestors sitting around a fire regaling one another with such stories.

- Traditional college juniors representing African-American, Hispanic, and Caucasian races and ethnicity.
- Learning theory: Cognitivist with Constructivist elements
- Instructional design model: Gagne's nine instructional events
- Resources: Computers, access to the Internet, handouts

Websites:

- Ancient Origins https://www.ancient-origins.net/google-earth
- Using Google Earth to locate Ancient Settlements: https://metaldetectingforum.com/showthread.php?t=221509

- Lost Mayan city FOUND using LASERS LIDAR, Ancient ruins found in jungle 2018https://video.search.yahoo.com/search/video;_ylt= AwrC5pbT9rVc 90kAM 6j7w8QF; _ ylu=X3oDMTB ncGdyMzQ0BHNlY wNzZWFy Y2gEdnRpZAM- ; _ylc=X1MDOTY 3ODEzMDcEX3IDMgRhY 3RuA2Nsaw RiY2sDYnY2OWxt MWU2 NzZmaSUy NmIlM0Qz JTI2cyUzRGF oBGNzcmNwdmlk A1NqWnQ2ak V3TGpHX 21UV3dYR09 aOGdKbk9E a3VNUUFBQUFDT mk3bWYEZnIDeWZ wLXQEZnIy A3NhLWdwB GdwcmlkA1hubm 5peUY5UkM2NDU 5T0tiQVV0ZE EEbXRlc 3RpZANud WxsBG5fcn. NsdAM2MA RuX3N1Z2c DMARvcmlnaW4Ddm lkZW8uc 2VhcmNoLnlha G9vLmNvbQRwb 3MDMARwcXN0 cgMEcHFzdHJsA wRxc3Ryb AM0NQRxd WVyeQNMSURBU iB0byBmaW5kIHRy

Table 11. Technology applied to archaeology: an overview

Nine Instructional Events by Gagne (1985, pp, 246-255)	
Preparation	
1. Gain attention	Begin: showing an excerpt from the use of LIDAR to strip away the Central American jungle to reveal an ancient city. Or, alternatively, show a movie clip featuring Indiana Jones finding the lost ark.
2. Inform about objectives	1. Describe the following technology and its use: a) Google Earth b) LIDAR c) Side scan sonar d) Ground penetrating radar 2. Find a potential archaeological site using Google Earth. 3. Conduct a WebQuest to find examples of technology applied to archaeology.
3. Recall of prior knowledge	Imagine the excitement of finding a lost city and beginning an excavation of it. This is a more precise undertaking than that of years gone by, of Schliemann, Carter, and others of like fame.
Instruction & Practice	
4. Present material	Break into two groups. Group one analyzes uses Google Earth to find a site of potential interest for further exploration. Group two analyzes the technology available to archaeologists in their search for traces of lost civilizations and ancient structures.
5. Provide Guidance	Walk among the groups to monitor their progress and their ideas.
6. Elicit performance	Have each group present their findings to the class at large.
7. Provide feedback	Provide feedback about their conclusions, their work as a team, and their presentation
Assignment & Transfer	
8. Assess performance	Assign grades in conjunction with peer grades
9. Enhance retention & transfer	Recap the lesson with a summary that includes a moral to the tale: "We are generally curious about the past to the extent that we try to find evidence of ancient civilizations and structures. What governs this urge?"

YWNlcyBvZiBh bmNpZW50IGN pdmlsaXphdGlvbn MEdF9zdG1w AzE1NTU0Mjky NjUEdnRlc3R pZANudWxs? gprid=Xnnniy F9RC6459OKb AUtdA&pvid= SjZt6jEwLjG_ mTWwX GOZ8gJn ODkuMQAAAACN i7mf&p=LIDAR+to+find +traces+of+ancient+civilizat ions&ei= UTF-8&fr2=p%3 As%2Cv% 3Av%2 Cm%3Asa& fr=yfp-t#id= 2&vid=bf7 b881bf7e 720c9907 b05a28e5ec 4c0&action=view

- Side-scan sonar used find plane wreckage off Jacksonville coasthttps:// www.news4jax.com/ video/side-scan-sonar- used-find-plane- wreckage -off-jacksonville- coast

Table 12. Topic 1: Nine instructional events by Gagne (1985, pp, 246-255)

Archaeology: Technology Applied to the Discipline **Topic/lesson 1: Technology** **LIDAR, Google Earth, side-scan sonar, and ground-penetrating radar are technological tools that archaeologists use in the exercise of their discipline.**	
Preparation	
1. Gain attention	Begin: show a video montage of LIDAR stripping away jungle overgrowth, Google Earth showing the outlines of an ancient civilization, side-scan sonar revealing a ship wreck on the floor of the ocean, and ground-penetrating radar revealing buried secrets invisible to the unaided eye. This could take only a few minutes.
2. Inform about objectives	1. Technology is giving archaeologists a new way to explore for the remains of ancient civilizations. What are some of these technologies? 2. How do they save time, money, and increase the probability of finding traces of ancient civilization?
3. Recall of prior knowledge	Can you tell me how radar works, sonar works? What are some examples from the natural world? Bats use echolocation as do dolphins.
Instruction & Practice	
4. Present material	Use the cognitivist approach with delivery by lecture and individual practice to apply the new knowledge. What does LIDAR mean? It means light detection and ranging. Sonar? Sound navigation and ranging. What is radar? Radio direction and ranging.
5. Provide Guidance	As you explain and illustrate the subject, ask questions to which you will respond with either affirmation of the correctness of the response or provide corrective instruction in the event of a wrong answer. End with a discussion about how these technologies help archaeologists as they practice their disciplines.
6. Elicit performance	After delivering the information, ask students to explain the words and describe the event in their own words.
7. Provide feedback	Comment on the explanations and ask questions of the class at large.
Assignment & Transfer	
8. Assess performance	Assign grades in conjunction with peer grades
9. Enhance retention & transfer	Recap the lesson with a summary that includes a moral to the tale, which is that these technologies expand the sensory capability of humans so that they can see beneath the jungle, beneath the sea, and beneath the earth.

Table 13. Topic 2: nine instructional events by Gagne (1985, pp, 246-255)

Archaeology: Technology Applied to the Discipline **Topic/lesson 2: Aerial Exploration** **Google Earth can help even amateur archaeologists find sites worthy of further investigation.**	
Preparation	
1. Gain attention	Begin: Show a video clip of aerial exploration in an airplane. This works best in the early morning or in the evening because of the shadows cast by the sun that can reveal trace marks of older civilizations. Then, go to a satellite view provided by Google Earth.
2. Inform about objectives	1. Aerial views help us to take advantage of the way light reveals subtle characteristics of the terrain. 2. Google Earth is available to anyone who has a computer and an Internet connection.
3. Recall of prior knowledge	Have you ever skimmed light over a surface to reveal details that were once hidden? Write a note on a pad and tear off the note that you have just written. Then, angle the sheet of paper that was under the note that you wrote, and you can see indentations of the note impressed upon the blank page.
Instruction & Practice	
4. Present material	Use the cognitivist approach with delivery by lecture and individual practice to apply the new knowledge. How can you take advantage of the light to find traces of objects that were obscured? One way is from an aerial perspective. You can obtain this by hot air balloon, an airplane, or a satellite.
5. Provide Guidance	As you explain and illustrate the subject, ask questions to which you will respond with either affirmation of the correctness of the response or provide corrective instruction in the event of a wrong answer. End with a discussion about how taking advantage of different lighting arrangements can help one to see traces of the past.
6. Elicit performance	After delivering the information, ask students to explain the words and describe the event in their own words.
7. Provide feedback	Comment on the explanations and ask questions of the class at large.
Assignment & Transfer	
8. Assess performance	Assign grades in conjunction with peer grades
9. Enhance retention & transfer	Recap the lesson with a summary that includes a moral to the tale, which is that Google Earth allows anyone who has a computer and an Internet connection to view the surface of the earth to seek the dim traces of now vanished civilizations.

Table 14. Topic 3: nine instructional events by Gagne (1985, pp, 246-255)

Archaeology: Technology Applied to the Discipline **Topic/lesson 3: The World Wide Web** **The Internet and a computer let you conduct a WebQuest to identify examples of the uses of archaeology technology**	
Preparation	
1. Gain attention	Begin: Show a video sequence of an individual conducting a WebQuest in search of various technologies that are applied to archaeology.
2. Inform about objectives	1. The Internet is a powerful tool with tremendous search capability. Let us put it to use. 2. The issue becomes one of finding the best search terms to use in our quest.
3. Recall of prior knowledge	The use of a search engine is very similar to an index. The index, in this case, being the entire Internet. The problem becomes one of finding the best term to use to explore the Internet. Think of the WebQuest as an exercise in using a vast index system.
Instruction & Practice	
4. Present material	Use the cognitivist approach with delivery by lecture and individual practice to apply the new knowledge. How can you find appropriate search terms in your quest? You can begin with a wide search and narrow it to a more specific search of terms. This can be done by using what is called Boolean logic, which is combining search terms with use of the words AND or OR and quotation marks.
5. Provide Guidance	As you explain and illustrate the subject, ask questions to which you will respond with either affirmation of the correctness of the response or provide corrective instruction in the event of a wrong answer. End with a discussion about how taking advantage of different search techniques and search engines.
6. Elicit performance	After delivering the information, ask students to explain the words and describe the event in their own words.
7. Provide feedback	Comment on the explanations and ask questions of the class at large.
Assignment & Transfer	
8. Assess performance	Assign grades in conjunction with peer grades
9. Enhance retention & transfer	Recap the lesson with a summary that includes a moral to the tale, which is that selection of general and specific search terms can make a significant difference in the productivity of your WebQuests.

- Ancient Viking ship found buried just 20 inches below ground on Norwegian farmland https://www.aol.com/article/news/2018/10/16/ancient-viking-ship-found-buried-just-20-inches-below-ground-on-norwegian-farmland/23563011/

REFERENCES

Gagné, R. M. (1985). *The conditions of learning and theory of instruction* (4th ed.). New York, NY: Holt, Rinehart, and Winston.

Hunt the Devil. (n.d.). Retrieved from https://huntthedevil.wordpress.com/2015/07/07/because-youre-here/

The Abolition Project. (2009). *William Wilberforce (1759-1833): The Politician.* Retrieved from http://abolition.e2bn.org/people_24.html

Williams, C. W. (2003). *History of Jones County, Georgia 1807-1907: Memorial edition.* Fernandina Beach, FL: Wolfe Publishing.

Appendix

APPENDIX A

Table 1. Learning theories by families and models within families

Model Family	Models
Paradigms	Behaviorism • Cognitivism • Constructivism • Design-Based • Humanism • 21st Century Skills
Constructivist, social and situational theories	Constructivism Overview Anchored Instruction (Bransford) Cognitive Apprenticeship (Collins et al.) Cognitive Dissonance (Festinger) Communities of Practice (Lave and Wenger) Connectivism (Siemens, Downes) Discovery Learning (Bruner) Ecological Theory of Development (Bronfenbrenner) Multiliteracies (New London Group) Semiotics (deSaussure, Barthes, Bakhtin) Social Development Theory (Vygotsky) Problem-Based Learning (PBL) Situated Learning (Lave)
Descriptive & meta theories	Activity Theory (Vygotsky, Leont'ev, Luria, Engstrom, etc.) Actor-Network Theory (Latour, Callon) Bloom's Taxonomy (Bloom) Distributed Cognition (Hutchins) Social Network Analysis (Scott, Prell)
Child development theories	Attachment Theory (Bowlby) Cognitive Tools Theory (Egan) Object Relations Theory (Klein) Montessori Method (Montessori) Separation-Individuation Theory of Child Development (Mahler)

continued on following page

Appendix

Table 1. Continued

Model Family	Models
Mental models	Backup Systems (Redundancy) Chaos Theory Confirmation Bias (Wason) Feedback Loops Inversion Law of Diminishing Returns Law of Large Numbers Network Effects Occam's Razor Pareto Principle Prisoner's Dilemma Scarcity Social Proof Tragedy of the Commons Transformative Learning
Behaviorist theories	Behaviorism Overview Classical Conditioning (Pavlov) GOMS Model (Card, Moran, and Newell) Operant Conditioning (Skinner) Psychological Behaviorism (Staats) Social Learning Theory (Albert Bandura)
Motivation and humanist theories	Humanism Overview ARCS Model of Motivational Design (Keller) Emotional Intelligence (Goleman) Experiential Learning (Kolb) Flow (Csikszentmihalyi) Grit (Duckworth, Matthews, Kelly, Peterson) Intrinsically Motivating Instruction (Malone) Maslow's Hierarchy of Needs (Maslow) Positive Psychology / PERMA Theory (Seligman) Self-Determination Theory (Deci and Ryan)
Identity theories	Erikson's Stages of Development (Erik Erikson) Identity Status Theory (Marcia) Mindset: Fixed vs. Growth Mindset (Dweck) Narcissism (Kernberg) Self-Perception Theory (Bem) Self-Theories: Entity and Incremental Theory (Dweck) Social Identity Theory (Tajfel, Turner) Stereotype Threat (Steele)
Miscellaneous learning theories and models	Affordance Theory (Gibson) Andragogy – Adult Learning Theory (Knowles) Flipped Classrooms Model of Hierarchical Complexity Multiple Intelligences Theory (Gardner) Systems Thinking 21st Century Skills (P21 and Others)
Guides, reviews, and learning tools	Cospaces: Creating Virtual Reality for the Classroom Card Game Toolkit: Create Educational Card Games Explore Learning: Interactive Gizmos and Simulations Flipgrid: Video Discussion Tool Maker Spaces for Education Mind Maps (Concept Maps) in the Classroom Tools to Teach Coding and Computer Science Robot Turtles Review: Coding Game for Kids Icebreakers Guide: Activities for the Classroom Ed Tech Guides

continued on following page

Table 1. Continued

Model Family	Models
Cognitivist theories	Cognitivism Overview Attribution Theory (Weiner) Cognitive Load Theory (Sweller) Cognitive Theory of Multimedia Learning (Mayer) Elaboration Theory (Reigeluth) Expertise Theory (Ericsson, Gladwell) Functional Context Theory (Sticht) Gestalt Theory (von Ehrenfels) Information Processing Theory Metacognition (Flavell) Situated Cognition (Brown, Collins & Duguid) Stage Theory of Cognitive Development (Piaget) Theory of Mind, Empathy, Mindblindness (Premack, Woodruff, Perner, Wimmer)
Design theories and models	Design-Based Research Overview ADDIE Model of Instructional Design ARCS Model of Motivational Design (Keller) Backward Design Elaboration Theory (Reigeluth) Learner-Centered Design (Soloway, Guzdian, Hay) Multimodality (Kress) SWOT Analysis Tool
Media and technology theories	Digital Citizenship Dopamine, Games and Motivation Educational Robotics and Constructionism (Papert) E-Learning Theory (Mayer, Sweller, Moreno) Game Reward Systems Gamification in Education Online Collaborative Learning (Harasim) Online Disinhibition Effect (Suler) Uses and Gratification Theory

Adapted from the listing provided at https://www.learning-theories.com/ (David, 2017).

David L, "Summaries of Learning Theories and Models," in Learning Theories, January 24, 2018, https://www.learning-theories.com/.

APPENDIX B

Table 2. Most common instructional design models

Model	Description
ADDIE	• Florida State University created the ADDIE Model for the U.S. Military in the 1970s ADDIE is an acronym for a process to develop courses. development process. The ADDIE Model generally consists of five interrelated phases—Analysis, Design, Development, Implementation, and Evaluation. The ADDIE Model represents a flexible guideline for building effective training and instructional materials ("Instructional Design Models"(n. d.), para. 2)."
SAM (successive approximation model)	SAM is a different approach to the development of instructional design products that address the performance need through iterations, repeated small steps, rather than with perfectly executed giant steps. SAM challenges the notion of moving through a linear process (like ADDIE) from Analysis to Evaluation as an effective strategy for designing learning events intending to produce greater performance. SAM addresses the roadblocks we all face (product quality, meeting timelines and budgets, and managing SMEs). Most importantly, SAM is an agile e-learning development process built specifically for the creation of performance-driven learning. Below are the core phases: Preparation: Instead of starting with a long, drawn-out evaluation of the existing or "needed" content, SAM starts with the preparation phase—where you gather information and get all the background knowledge. This is intended to be a very quick phase. Iterative Design: This phase begins with the Savvy Start, the initial collaborative brainstorming meeting that establishes the foundation for a successful project. The Savvy Start focuses primarily on performance and will serve as the project kickoff meeting and the main environment for all project team members to converse. Throughout the Savvy Start and the Iterative Design Phase, your team will be rotating through design, prototype, and review. Iterative Development: Much like the Iterative Design Phase, in the Iterative Development Phase your team will rotate through development, implementation, and evaluation. You'll start with your design proof, moving to Alpha and Beta, before finally rolling out the Gold. As the instructional product is being developed, you continually analyze and evaluate, so that at any point if a change needs to occur, it can happen quickly and limit any risk of the project moving out of budget or time." Source: www.alleninteractions.com
Action Mapping	"Action Mapping is a quick, effective, and visual way to design compelling learning experiences for instructional products including eLearning, simulations, and in person training events. It is called action mapping because it helps change what people do, not just what they know. It helps to design action-packed materials that are 100% dedicated to improving business performance. Additionally, it can keep stakeholders from adding extraneous information." Source: www.blog.cathy-moore.com"
Learning Circle Framework	Instructional Design Central (IDC) has created a three-phase, easy-to-follow framework to rapidly build and present your learning design strategy—The Learning Circle Framework™. The Learning Circle Framework™ is founded on modern learning design and product development principles. See an overview of The Learning Circle Framework™

continued on following page

Table 2. Continued

Model	Description
Merrill's First Principles of Instruction	"Many current instructional design models suggest that the most effective learning environments are those that are problem-based and involve the student in four distinct phases of learning: (1) activation of prior experience, (2) demonstration of skills, (3) application of skills, and (4) integration of these skills into real world activities. Figure 2 below illustrates these five ideas. Much instructional practice concentrates primarily on phase 2 and ignores the other phases in this cycle of learning."
Gagné's 9 Events of Instruction	"Robert Gagné is considered to be the foremost contributor to the systematic approach to instructional design and training. Gagne and his followers are known as behaviorists, and their focus is on the outcomes (or behaviors) resulting from training. Gagné's book, The Conditions of Learning, identified the mental conditions for learning. Gagné created a nine-step process called the events of instruction, which correlate to and address the conditions of learning. See the nine events of instruction below: Source: www.edutechwiki.unige.ch"
Bloom's Taxonomy	"In 1956, Benjamin Bloom headed a group of educational psychologists who developed a classification of levels of intellectual behavior important in learning. Bloom found that over 95% of the test questions students encounter require them to think only at the lowest possible level...the recall of information. Bloom identified six levels within the cognitive domain, from the simple recall or recognition of facts, as the lowest level, through increasingly more complex and abstract mental levels, to the highest order which is classified as evaluation."
Dick and Carey Model	"Another well-known instructional design model is The Dick and Carey Systems Approach Model. The model was originally published in 1978 by Walter Dick and Lou Carey in their book entitled The Systematic Design of Instruction. Dick and Carey made a significant contribution to the instructional design field by championing a systems view of instruction as opposed to viewing instruction as a sum of isolated parts. The model addresses instruction as an entire system, focusing on the interrelationship between context, content, learning, and instruction. According to Dick and Carey, "Components such as the instructor, learners, materials, instructional activities, delivery system, and learning and performance environments interact with each other and work together to bring about the desired student learning outcomes".
Kemp Instructional Design Model	"The Jerold Kemp instructional design method and model defines nine different components of instructional design and at the same time adopts a continuous implementation/evaluation model. Kemp adopts a wide view, the oval shape of his model conveys that the design and development process is a continuous cycle that requires constant planning, design, development, and assessment to insure effective instruction. The model is systemic and nonlinear and seems to encourage designers to work in all areas as appropriate (Steven McGriff). The model is particularly useful for developing instructional programs that blend technology, pedagogy and content to deliver effective, inclusive (reliable) and efficient learning. Source: www.edutechwiki.unige.ch"
Kirkpatrick's Four Levels of Training Evaluation	"The Kirkpatrick Model is the worldwide standard for evaluating the effectiveness of training. It considers the value of any type of training, formal or informal, across four levels:
	• Level 1 Reaction evaluates how participants respond to the training. • Level 2 Learning measures if they actually learned the material. • Level 3 Behavior considers if they are using what they learned on the job. • Level 4 Results evaluates if the training positively impacted the organization. • Source, http://www.kirkpatrickpartners.com"

The above material was adapted from Instructional Design Models (n. d.). Retrieved from https://www.instructionaldesigncentral.com/instructionaldesignmodels

REFERENCES

David, L. (2017). *Learning theories in plain English*. Retrieved from https://www.learning-theories.com/

Instructional Design Models. (n.d.). Retrieved from http://www.instructionaldesign.org/models/

Related Readings

To continue IGI Global's long-standing tradition of advancing innovation through emerging research, please find below a compiled list of recommended IGI Global book chapters and journal articles in the areas of massively open online courses, higher education, and learning analytics. These related readings will provide additional information and guidance to further enrich your knowledge and assist you with your own research.

Ackerman, G. L. (2018). Open Source Online Learning in Rural Communities. In I. Bouchrika, N. Harrati, & P. Vu (Eds.), *Learner Experience and Usability in Online Education* (pp. 61–84). Hershey, PA: IGI Global. doi:10.4018/978-1-5225-4206-3.ch003

Alharbi, H., & Sandhu, K. (2018). Robust Data Findings of E-Learning Analytics Recommender Systems and Their Impact on System Adoption for Student Experiences. *International Journal of Organizational and Collective Intelligence*, *8*(3), 1–12. doi:10.4018/IJOCI.2018070101

Alharbi, H., & Sandhu, K. (2019). New Discoveries for User Acceptance of E-Learning Analytics Recommender Systems in Saudi Arabia. *International Journal of Innovation in the Digital Economy*, *10*(1), 31–42. doi:10.4018/IJIDE.2019010103

Alharbi, H., & Sandhu, K. (2019). New Empirical Data Findings for Student Experiences of E-Learning analytics Recommender Systems and their Impact on System Adoption. *International Journal of Innovation in the Digital Economy*, *10*(2), 54–63. doi:10.4018/IJIDE.2019040104

Almjeld, J. (2017). Getting "Girly" Online: The Case for Gendering Online Spaces. In E. Monske & K. Blair (Eds.), *Handbook of Research on Writing and Composing in the Age of MOOCs* (pp. 87–105). Hershey, PA: IGI Global. doi:10.4018/978-1-5225-1718-4.ch006

Alomyan, H. (2018). Issues in Web-Based Learning. In I. Bouchrika, N. Harrati, & P. Vu (Eds.), *Learner Experience and Usability in Online Education* (pp. 235–255). Hershey, PA: IGI Global. doi:10.4018/978-1-5225-4206-3.ch009

Ammenwerth, E., Hackl, W. O., Hoerbst, A., & Felderer, M. (2019). Indicators for Cooperative, Online-Based Learning and Their Role in Quality Management of Online Learning. In M. Boboc & S. Koç (Eds.), *Student-Centered Virtual Learning Environments in Higher Education* (pp. 1–20). Hershey, PA: IGI Global. doi:10.4018/978-1-5225-5769-2.ch001

Babb, J. (2017). Reshaping Institutional Mission: OWI and Writing Program Administration. In E. Monske & K. Blair (Eds.), *Handbook of Research on Writing and Composing in the Age of MOOCs* (pp. 202–215). Hershey, PA: IGI Global. doi:10.4018/978-1-5225-1718-4.ch013

Bader, J. D., & Lowenthal, P. R. (2018). Using Visual Design to Improve the Online Learning Experience: A Synthesis of Research on Aesthetics. In I. Bouchrika, N. Harrati, & P. Vu (Eds.), *Learner Experience and Usability in Online Education* (pp. 1–35). Hershey, PA: IGI Global. doi:10.4018/978-1-5225-4206-3.ch001

Baker, N. L., & Buck, E. H. (2017). Conducting Programmatic Assessments of Online Writing Instruction: CCCC's OWI Principles in Practice. In E. Monske & K. Blair (Eds.), *Handbook of Research on Writing and Composing in the Age of MOOCs* (pp. 385–405). Hershey, PA: IGI Global. doi:10.4018/978-1-5225-1718-4.ch023

Borgman, J. C. (2017). The Online Writing Program Administrator (OWPA): Maintaining a Brand in the Age of MOOCs. In E. Monske & K. Blair (Eds.), *Handbook of Research on Writing and Composing in the Age of MOOCs* (pp. 188–201). Hershey, PA: IGI Global. doi:10.4018/978-1-5225-1718-4.ch012

Bourelle, T., & Hewett, B. L. (2017). Training Instructors to Teach Multimodal Composition in Online Courses. In E. Monske & K. Blair (Eds.), *Handbook of Research on Writing and Composing in the Age of MOOCs* (pp. 348–369). Hershey, PA: IGI Global. doi:10.4018/978-1-5225-1718-4.ch021

Branson, T. (2017). Problematic Partnerships: An Analysis of Three Composition MOOCs Funded by the Gates Foundation. In E. Monske & K. Blair (Eds.), *Handbook of Research on Writing and Composing in the Age of MOOCs* (pp. 169–187). Hershey, PA: IGI Global. doi:10.4018/978-1-5225-1718-4.ch011

Browning, L. G., & Dorner, L. M. (2018). Missing Opportunity?: Rural School Board Members and Data Use. In E. Mense & M. Crain-Dorough (Eds.), *Data Leadership for K-12 Schools in a Time of Accountability* (pp. 184–205). Hershey, PA: IGI Global. doi:10.4018/978-1-5225-3188-3.ch010

Cocquyt, C., Diep, A. N., Zhu, C., De Greef, M., & Vanwing, T. (2019). Towards Blended Learning Designs Fostering Adults' Social Capital: What Do Empirical Findings Reveal? In E. Ossiannilsson (Ed.), *Ubiquitous Inclusive Learning in a Digital Era* (pp. 55–80). Hershey, PA: IGI Global. doi:10.4018/978-1-5225-6292-4.ch003

Colby, R. (2017). A Typology of MOOCS. In E. Monske & K. Blair (Eds.), *Handbook of Research on Writing and Composing in the Age of MOOCs* (pp. 1–16). Hershey, PA: IGI Global. doi:10.4018/978-1-5225-1718-4.ch001

Colby, R. S. (2017). Using Online Writing Communities to Teach Writing MOOCs. In E. Monske & K. Blair (Eds.), *Handbook of Research on Writing and Composing in the Age of MOOCs* (pp. 317–330). Hershey, PA: IGI Global. doi:10.4018/978-1-5225-1718-4.ch019

Crain-Dorough, M., & Elder, A. C. (2018). Making Research Methods Instruction Relevant for Prospective Principals: The Development of Data Literacy for Effective Data Use. In E. Mense & M. Crain-Dorough (Eds.), *Data Leadership for K-12 Schools in a Time of Accountability* (pp. 260–283). Hershey, PA: IGI Global. doi:10.4018/978-1-5225-3188-3.ch013

Cypret-Mahach, R. (2018). Transformational Shifts of Pedagogy Through Professional Development, Essential Questions, and Self-Directed Learning. In F. Giuseffi (Ed.), *Emerging Self-Directed Learning Strategies in the Digital Age* (pp. 160–178). Hershey, PA: IGI Global. doi:10.4018/978-1-5225-3465-5.ch008

Dash, A. R., & Patra, M. R. (2018). Ensuring Quality of Web Portals Through Accessibility Analysis. In I. Bouchrika, N. Harrati, & P. Vu (Eds.), *Learner Experience and Usability in Online Education* (pp. 194–234). Hershey, PA: IGI Global. doi:10.4018/978-1-5225-4206-3.ch008

Galaige, J., & Torrisi-Steele, G. (2019). Unpacking the 'Learning' in Student-Facing Analytics: Metacognition and the Zone of Proximal Development. *International Journal of Adult Vocational Education and Technology*, *10*(1), 1–12. doi:10.4018/IJAVET.2019010101

Giesteira, B., & Pereira, E. (2018). HCI4D Guidelines for Interactive Content. In R. Queirós (Ed.), *Emerging Trends, Techniques, and Tools for Massive Open Online Course (MOOC) Management* (pp. 49–77). Hershey, PA: IGI Global. doi:10.4018/978-1-5225-5011-2.ch003

Gomes, M. A., Sharma, R. C., Matta, A. E., & Robatto, L. (2019). Three Dimensional (3D) Simulation for Ubiquitous and Inclusive Learning in a Digital Era. In E. Ossiannilsson (Ed.), *Ubiquitous Inclusive Learning in a Digital Era* (pp. 228–251). Hershey, PA: IGI Global. doi:10.4018/978-1-5225-6292-4.ch010

Grant-Smith, D., Donnet, T., Macaulay, J., & Chapman, R. (2019). Principles and Practices for Enhanced Visual Design in Virtual Learning Environments: Do Looks Matter in Student Engagement? In M. Boboc & S. Koç (Eds.), *Student-Centered Virtual Learning Environments in Higher Education* (pp. 103–133). Hershey, PA: IGI Global. doi:10.4018/978-1-5225-5769-2.ch005

Hambrock, H. B., & Richter, R. G. (2019). A Pedagogical Approach Towards Curating Mobile Apps in an Educational Context. In E. Ossiannilsson (Ed.), *Ubiquitous Inclusive Learning in a Digital Era* (pp. 81–106). Hershey, PA: IGI Global. doi:10.4018/978-1-5225-6292-4.ch004

Hayag, M. R. Jr. (2018). Learning Analytics: Application on Curriculum Design and Assessment. In M. Kumar Singh, Z. Zerihun, & N. Singh (Eds.), *Impact of Learning Analytics on Curriculum Design and Student Performance* (pp. 113–124). Hershey, PA: IGI Global. doi:10.4018/978-1-5225-5369-4.ch008

Hayes, S. D., & Lee, C. G. (2018). The Principal as a Data-Driven Instructional Leader: Using PLCs to Improve Teaching and Learning. In E. Mense & M. Crain-Dorough (Eds.), *Data Leadership for K-12 Schools in a Time of Accountability* (pp. 76–97). Hershey, PA: IGI Global. doi:10.4018/978-1-5225-3188-3.ch005

Henry, T. P. (2017). What's a "Technician" to Do?: Theorizing and Articulating MOOC Maintenance Concerns. In E. Monske & K. Blair (Eds.), *Handbook of Research on Writing and Composing in the Age of MOOCs* (pp. 216–231). Hershey, PA: IGI Global. doi:10.4018/978-1-5225-1718-4.ch014

Herring, T. (2018). Data Dissemination Practices of Elementary School Principals. In E. Mense & M. Crain-Dorough (Eds.), *Data Leadership for K-12 Schools in a Time of Accountability* (pp. 19–38). Hershey, PA: IGI Global. doi:10.4018/978-1-5225-3188-3.ch002

Hewett, B. L., & Warnock, S. (2017). Writing MOOEEs?: Reconsidering MOOCs in Light of the OWI Principles. In E. Monske & K. Blair (Eds.), *Handbook of Research on Writing and Composing in the Age of MOOCs* (pp. 17–38). Hershey, PA: IGI Global. doi:10.4018/978-1-5225-1718-4.ch002

Hill, V. (2017). Digital Citizens as Writers: New Literacies and New Responsibilities. In E. Monske & K. Blair (Eds.), *Handbook of Research on Writing and Composing in the Age of MOOCs* (pp. 56–74). Hershey, PA: IGI Global. doi:10.4018/978-1-5225-1718-4.ch004

Hood, N., & Littlejohn, A. (2019). Disruptive Democratisers?: The Complexities and Incongruities of Scale, Diversity and Personalisation in MOOCs. In E. Ossiannilsson (Ed.), *Ubiquitous Inclusive Learning in a Digital Era* (pp. 1–28). Hershey, PA: IGI Global. doi:10.4018/978-1-5225-6292-4.ch001

Howard, L. (2017). A (Critical) Distance: Contingent Labor, MOOCs, and Teaching Online. In E. Monske & K. Blair (Eds.), *Handbook of Research on Writing and Composing in the Age of MOOCs* (pp. 232–253). Hershey, PA: IGI Global. doi:10.4018/978-1-5225-1718-4.ch015

Hsu, Y., Meyen, E. L., & Lee, Y. (2019). Understanding Emotional Analytics for Student Engagement: An Instructional Design Perspective. In M. Boboc & S. Koç (Eds.), *Student-Centered Virtual Learning Environments in Higher Education* (pp. 70–102). Hershey, PA: IGI Global. doi:10.4018/978-1-5225-5769-2.ch004

Irwin, L. H., & Reames, E. H. (2018). Towards Partnerships for Student Success: Teacher Collaboration in Data Analysis and Common Formative Assessment Systems. In E. Mense & M. Crain-Dorough (Eds.), *Data Leadership for K-12 Schools in a Time of Accountability* (pp. 140–156). Hershey, PA: IGI Global. doi:10.4018/978-1-5225-3188-3.ch008

Jenkins, P. (2017). Arguing for Proactivity: Talking Points for Owning Accessibility in Online Writing Instruction. In E. Monske & K. Blair (Eds.), *Handbook of Research on Writing and Composing in the Age of MOOCs* (pp. 106–122). Hershey, PA: IGI Global. doi:10.4018/978-1-5225-1718-4.ch007

Johnson, M. L. (2018). Empowering Educators to Make Data-Informed Decisions: A District's Journey of Effective Data Use. In E. Mense & M. Crain-Dorough (Eds.), *Data Leadership for K-12 Schools in a Time of Accountability* (pp. 158–183). Hershey, PA: IGI Global. doi:10.4018/978-1-5225-3188-3.ch009

Johnston, E. A., Olivas, G. W., Steele, P., Smith, C., & Bailey, L. W. (2019). Virtual Reality Pedagogical Considerations in Learning Environments. In M. Boboc & S. Koç (Eds.), *Student-Centered Virtual Learning Environments in Higher Education* (pp. 21–39). Hershey, PA: IGI Global. doi:10.4018/978-1-5225-5769-2.ch002

Jurado, F., & Rodriguez, P. (2018). The Learning Style of Gamers: Exploring a Multidimensional Profile Aimed at Gamifying MOOCs. In R. Queirós (Ed.), *Emerging Trends, Techniques, and Tools for Massive Open Online Course (MOOC) Management* (pp. 106–129). Hershey, PA: IGI Global. doi:10.4018/978-1-5225-5011-2.ch005

Kashtwari, D. M., & Wani, Z. A. (2019). MOOCs: The Indian Journey So Far. In E. Ossiannilsson (Ed.), *Ubiquitous Inclusive Learning in a Digital Era* (pp. 29–54). Hershey, PA: IGI Global. doi:10.4018/978-1-5225-6292-4.ch002

Khan, M. S., Nambobi, M., & Ali, M. S. (2018). MOOCs in TVET Sectors of Developing Countries: Benefits, Possibilities, and Challenges. In F. Giuseffi (Ed.), *Emerging Self-Directed Learning Strategies in the Digital Age* (pp. 22–47). Hershey, PA: IGI Global. doi:10.4018/978-1-5225-3465-5.ch003

Lancaster, S. J., & Topper, A. (2019). Designing and Implementing a Student-Centered Online Graduate Program: A Case Study in a College of Education. In M. Boboc & S. Koç (Eds.), *Student-Centered Virtual Learning Environments in Higher Education* (pp. 157–184). Hershey, PA: IGI Global. doi:10.4018/978-1-5225-5769-2.ch007

Lin, L. (2018). Student Learning and Engagement in a Blended Environment: A Mixed Methods Study. In I. Bouchrika, N. Harrati, & P. Vu (Eds.), *Learner Experience and Usability in Online Education* (pp. 256–269). Hershey, PA: IGI Global. doi:10.4018/978-1-5225-4206-3.ch010

Liu, M., Pardo, A., & Liu, L. (2017). Using Learning Analytics to Support Engagement in Collaborative Writing. *International Journal of Distance Education Technologies, 15*(4), 79–98. doi:10.4018/IJDET.2017100105

Liu, S., Hu, Z., Peng, X., Liu, Z., Cheng, H. N., & Sun, J. (2017). Mining Learning Behavioral Patterns of Students by Sequence Analysis in Cloud Classroom. *International Journal of Distance Education Technologies, 15*(1), 15–27. doi:10.4018/IJDET.2017010102

Liu, S., Ni, C., Liu, Z., Peng, X., & Cheng, H. N. (2017). Mining Individual Learning Topics in Course Reviews Based on Author Topic Model. *International Journal of Distance Education Technologies, 15*(3), 1–14. doi:10.4018/IJDET.2017070101

Long, J. D. (2018). The Intersection of Andragogy and Dissertation Writing: How Andragogy Can Improve the Process. In F. Giuseffi (Ed.), *Emerging Self-Directed Learning Strategies in the Digital Age* (pp. 81-108). Hershey, PA: IGI Global. doi:10.4018/978-1-5225-3465-5.ch005

Luo, T., & Baaki, J. (2019). Scaffolding Problem-Solving and Instructional Design Processes: Engaging Students in Reflection-in-Action and External Representations in Three Online Courses. In M. Boboc & S. Koç (Eds.), *Student-Centered Virtual Learning Environments in Higher Education* (pp. 40–69). Hershey, PA: IGI Global. doi:10.4018/978-1-5225-5769-2.ch003

Lusta, A. F. (2018). Investigating MOOC Arabic Learners' Motivation in Language Online Courses (MOOCs). In R. Queirós (Ed.), *Emerging Trends, Techniques, and Tools for Massive Open Online Course (MOOC) Management* (pp. 156–179). Hershey, PA: IGI Global. doi:10.4018/978-1-5225-5011-2.ch007

Mahmoudi, L., & Gronseth, S. (2019). Video-Based Discussion: Promoting Presence Through Interactions in Online Higher Education Courses. In E. Ossiannilsson (Ed.), *Ubiquitous Inclusive Learning in a Digital Era* (pp. 128–153). Hershey, PA: IGI Global. doi:10.4018/978-1-5225-6292-4.ch006

Malik, N. (2018). Learning Analytics in the Perspective of Enhancing Students' Performance. In M. Kumar Singh, Z. Zerihun, & N. Singh (Eds.), *Impact of Learning Analytics on Curriculum Design and Student Performance* (pp. 125–141). Hershey, PA: IGI Global. doi:10.4018/978-1-5225-5369-4.ch009

Mariano, G. J., & Batchelor, K. (2018). The Role of Metacogntion and Knowledge Transfer in Self-Directed Learning. In F. Giuseffi (Ed.), *Emerging Self-Directed Learning Strategies in the Digital Age* (pp. 141–159). Hershey, PA: IGI Global. doi:10.4018/978-1-5225-3465-5.ch007

Martini, R. H., & Webster, T. (2017). What Online Writing Spaces Afford Us in the Age of Campus Carry, "Wall-Building," and Orlando's Pulse Tragedy. In E. Monske & K. Blair (Eds.), *Handbook of Research on Writing and Composing in the Age of MOOCs* (pp. 278–293). Hershey, PA: IGI Global. doi:10.4018/978-1-5225-1718-4.ch017

McEachern, R. W. (2017). Challenging Evaluation: The Complexity of Grading Writing in Hybrid MOOCs. In E. Monske & K. Blair (Eds.), *Handbook of Research on Writing and Composing in the Age of MOOCs* (pp. 370–384). Hershey, PA: IGI Global. doi:10.4018/978-1-5225-1718-4.ch022

Mense, E. G., Griggs, D. M., & Shanks, J. N. (2018). School Leaders in a Time of Accountability and Data Use: Preparing Our Future School Leaders in Leadership Preparation Programs. In E. Mense & M. Crain-Dorough (Eds.), *Data Leadership for K-12 Schools in a Time of Accountability* (pp. 235–259). Hershey, PA: IGI Global. doi:10.4018/978-1-5225-3188-3.ch012

Mihăeş, L. C., & Epure, M. (2019). Insights Into University-Business Cooperation in the Information Society: A Romanian Project for Higher Education. In E. Ossiannilsson (Ed.), *Ubiquitous Inclusive Learning in a Digital Era* (pp. 199–227). Hershey, PA: IGI Global. doi:10.4018/978-1-5225-6292-4.ch009

Miteva, D., Stefanov, K., & Stefanova, E. (2017). e-Analytics for e-Learning. *International Journal of Human Capital and Information Technology Professionals*, *8*(4), 1–13. doi:10.4018/IJHCITP.2017100101

Mouri, K., Ren, Z., Uosaki, N., & Yin, C. (2019). Analyzing Learning Patterns Based on Log Data from Digital Textbooks. *International Journal of Distance Education Technologies*, *17*(1), 1–14. doi:10.4018/IJDET.2019010101

Murray, R. W., & Murray, M. A. (2018). Behind the Scenes of Data-Driven Leadership: Intentionality of Leadership. In E. Mense & M. Crain-Dorough (Eds.), *Data Leadership for K-12 Schools in a Time of Accountability* (pp. 1–18). Hershey, PA: IGI Global. doi:10.4018/978-1-5225-3188-3.ch001

Nobre, A., Mallmann, E. M., Nobre, V., & Mazzardo, M. D. (2018). MOOC and OER: Identity Management. In R. Queirós (Ed.), *Emerging Trends, Techniques, and Tools for Massive Open Online Course (MOOC) Management* (pp. 1–23). Hershey, PA: IGI Global. doi:10.4018/978-1-5225-5011-2.ch001

Novak, J. I. (2019). Self-Directed Learning in the Age of Open Source, Open Hardware and 3D Printing. In E. Ossiannilsson (Ed.), *Ubiquitous Inclusive Learning in a Digital Era* (pp. 154–178). Hershey, PA: IGI Global. doi:10.4018/978-1-5225-6292-4.ch007

Nunes, F. B., Zunguze, M. C., Hannel, K., Antunes, F. F., Franco, S. R., & De Lima, J. V. (2018). Analysis of Users in an Immersive Environment for Teaching Science. In I. Bouchrika, N. Harrati, & P. Vu (Eds.), *Learner Experience and Usability in Online Education* (pp. 149–173). Hershey, PA: IGI Global. doi:10.4018/978-1-5225-4206-3.ch006

Odom, S., & Lindsey, L. (2017). Hacking the Lecture: Transgressive Praxis and Presence Using Online Video. In E. Monske & K. Blair (Eds.), *Handbook of Research on Writing and Composing in the Age of MOOCs* (pp. 331–347). Hershey, PA: IGI Global. doi:10.4018/978-1-5225-1718-4.ch020

Önaçan, M. B., Uluağ, M., Önel, T., & Medeni, T. D. (2018). Selection of Plagiarism Detection Software and Its Integration Into Moodle for Universities: An Example of Open Source Software Use in Developing Countries. In R. Queirós (Ed.), *Emerging Trends, Techniques, and Tools for Massive Open Online Course (MOOC) Management* (pp. 239–258). Hershey, PA: IGI Global. doi:10.4018/978-1-5225-5011-2.ch010

Orlando, M., & Howard, L. (2018). Setting the Stage for Success in an Online Learning Environment. In F. Giuseffi (Ed.), *Emerging Self-Directed Learning Strategies in the Digital Age* (pp. 1–9). Hershey, PA: IGI Global. doi:10.4018/978-1-5225-3465-5.ch001

Ossiannilsson, E. (2018). Increasing Access, Social Inclusion, and Quality Through Mobile Learning. *International Journal of Advanced Pervasive and Ubiquitous Computing*, *10*(4), 29–44. doi:10.4018/IJAPUC.2018100103

Oswal, S. K. (2017). MOOCs in the Global Context. In E. Monske & K. Blair (Eds.), *Handbook of Research on Writing and Composing in the Age of MOOCs* (pp. 39–55). Hershey, PA: IGI Global. doi:10.4018/978-1-5225-1718-4.ch003

Overstreet, M. (2017). Principled/Digital: Composition's "Ethics of Attunement" and the Writing MOOC. In E. Monske & K. Blair (Eds.), *Handbook of Research on Writing and Composing in the Age of MOOCs* (pp. 75–86). Hershey, PA: IGI Global. doi:10.4018/978-1-5225-1718-4.ch005

Paneva-Marinova, D., & Pavlov, R. (2018). Improving Learner Experience Within Educational Nooks in Digital Libraries. In I. Bouchrika, N. Harrati, & P. Vu (Eds.), *Learner Experience and Usability in Online Education* (pp. 174–193). Hershey, PA: IGI Global. doi:10.4018/978-1-5225-4206-3.ch007

Pérez-Juárez, M. A., Antón-Rodríguez, M., Díaz-Pernas, F. J., Martínez-Zarzuela, M., & González-Ortega, D. (2018). An Analysis of the Possibilities of the Use of Technology for the Learning of Languages: From CSCL to Cloud Computing and MOOCs. In R. Queirós (Ed.), *Emerging Trends, Techniques, and Tools for Massive Open Online Course (MOOC) Management* (pp. 180–212). Hershey, PA: IGI Global. doi:10.4018/978-1-5225-5011-2.ch008

Petrosino, K. L. (2017). Developmental Writing and MOOCs: Reconsidering Access, Remediation, and Development in Large-Scale Online Writing Instruction. In E. Monske & K. Blair (Eds.), *Handbook of Research on Writing and Composing in the Age of MOOCs* (pp. 153–168). Hershey, PA: IGI Global. doi:10.4018/978-1-5225-1718-4.ch010

Quezada, T., Brunk-Chavez, B., & Posey, E. (2017). Connecting Writing Studies with Online Programs: UTEP's Graduate Technical and Professional Writing Certificate Program. In E. Monske & K. Blair (Eds.), *Handbook of Research on Writing and Composing in the Age of MOOCs* (pp. 123–136). Hershey, PA: IGI Global. doi:10.4018/978-1-5225-1718-4.ch008

Rajabi, E., & Greller, W. (2019). Exposing Social Data as Linked Data in Education. *International Journal on Semantic Web and Information Systems, 15*(2), 92–106. doi:10.4018/IJSWIS.2019040105

Rock, H. M. (2019). A Framework for Effective Online Professional Development. In M. Boboc & S. Koç (Eds.), *Student-Centered Virtual Learning Environments in Higher Education* (pp. 210–232). Hershey, PA: IGI Global. doi:10.4018/978-1-5225-5769-2.ch009

Rodrigues, R. L., Ramos, J. L., Silva, J. C., Dourado, R. A., & Gomes, A. S. (2019). Forecasting Students' Performance Through Self-Regulated Learning Behavioral Analysis. *International Journal of Distance Education Technologies, 17*(3), 52–74. doi:10.4018/IJDET.2019070104

Rysavy, M. D., Michalak, R., & Hunt, K. (2018). Information Literacy Education for First-Year Composition Students: A Case Study of Three Deployment Modes. In I. Bouchrika, N. Harrati, & P. Vu (Eds.), *Learner Experience and Usability in Online Education* (pp. 85–121). Hershey, PA: IGI Global. doi:10.4018/978-1-5225-4206-3.ch004

Sanchez-Gordon, S., & Luján-Mora, S. (2018). Lifecycle for MOOC Development and Management. In R. Queirós (Ed.), *Emerging Trends, Techniques, and Tools for Massive Open Online Course (MOOC) Management* (pp. 24–48). Hershey, PA: IGI Global. doi:10.4018/978-1-5225-5011-2.ch002

Sani-Bozkurt, S. (2019). Universal Design Principles and Technology-Supported Learning in the Digital Era: Assistive Technologies in Inclusive Learning. In E. Ossiannilsson (Ed.), *Ubiquitous Inclusive Learning in a Digital Era* (pp. 107–127). Hershey, PA: IGI Global. doi:10.4018/978-1-5225-6292-4.ch005

Schildkamp, K., & Poortman, C. L. (2018). Leadership to Support and Sustain Data Use in Data Teams. In E. Mense & M. Crain-Dorough (Eds.), *Data Leadership for K-12 Schools in a Time of Accountability* (pp. 98–118). Hershey, PA: IGI Global. doi:10.4018/978-1-5225-3188-3.ch006

Shanks, J. N. (2018). Establishing a Data Culture Using a Data-Driven Instructional System for School Improvement. In E. Mense & M. Crain-Dorough (Eds.), *Data Leadership for K-12 Schools in a Time of Accountability* (pp. 39–53). Hershey, PA: IGI Global. doi:10.4018/978-1-5225-3188-3.ch003

Shi, H., & Witte, M. M. (2018). Self-Directed Language Learning, Asian Cultural Influences, and the Teacher's Role. In F. Giuseffi (Ed.), *Emerging Self-Directed Learning Strategies in the Digital Age* (pp. 109–140). Hershey, PA: IGI Global. doi:10.4018/978-1-5225-3465-5.ch006

Shoukry, L., Konert, J., & Göbel, S. (2018). The Evaluation of Learner Experience in Serious Games. In I. Bouchrika, N. Harrati, & P. Vu (Eds.), *Learner Experience and Usability in Online Education* (pp. 122–148). Hershey, PA: IGI Global. doi:10.4018/978-1-5225-4206-3.ch005

Silva, J. C., Zambom, E., Rodrigues, R. L., Ramos, J. L., & de Souza, F. D. (2018). Effects of Learning Analytics on Students' Self-Regulated Learning in Flipped Classroom. *International Journal of Information and Communication Technology Education*, *14*(3), 91–107. doi:10.4018/IJICTE.2018070108

Singh, M. K. (2018). Challenges of Learning Analytics Execution in the Educational System. In M. Kumar Singh, Z. Zerihun, & N. Singh (Eds.), *Impact of Learning Analytics on Curriculum Design and Student Performance* (pp. 28–40). Hershey, PA: IGI Global. doi:10.4018/978-1-5225-5369-4.ch003

Singh, M. K. (2018). Implementation and Impact of Learning Analytics on Multifarious Educational Systems: Technique and Process. In M. Kumar Singh, Z. Zerihun, & N. Singh (Eds.), *Impact of Learning Analytics on Curriculum Design and Student Performance* (pp. 142–152). Hershey, PA: IGI Global. doi:10.4018/978-1-5225-5369-4.ch010

Singh, N. (2018). A Study on the Impact of Learning Analytics to Evaluate Students' Performance in Higher Education. In M. Kumar Singh, Z. Zerihun, & N. Singh (Eds.), *Impact of Learning Analytics on Curriculum Design and Student Performance* (pp. 19–27). Hershey, PA: IGI Global. doi:10.4018/978-1-5225-5369-4.ch002

Singh, N. (2018). Impact of Learning Analytics on the Assessment of a Curriculum-Based Test. In M. Kumar Singh, Z. Zerihun, & N. Singh (Eds.), *Impact of Learning Analytics on Curriculum Design and Student Performance* (pp. 56–70). Hershey, PA: IGI Global. doi:10.4018/978-1-5225-5369-4.ch005

Singh, R. P. (2018). Learning Analytics: Potential, Protection, and Privacy in the Educational System. In M. Kumar Singh, Z. Zerihun, & N. Singh (Eds.), *Impact of Learning Analytics on Curriculum Design and Student Performance* (pp. 1–18). Hershey, PA: IGI Global. doi:10.4018/978-1-5225-5369-4.ch001

Soares, F., & Lopes, A. P. (2018). M100S Project: Math MOOCs From Polytechnic of Porto – Development, Continuance, and Use. In R. Queirós (Ed.), *Emerging Trends, Techniques, and Tools for Massive Open Online Course (MOOC) Management* (pp. 213–238). Hershey, PA: IGI Global. doi:10.4018/978-1-5225-5011-2.ch009

Steffen, V. T. (2017). Contact and Interactivity in Televised Learning: 15 Years Later. In E. Monske & K. Blair (Eds.), *Handbook of Research on Writing and Composing in the Age of MOOCs* (pp. 137–152). Hershey, PA: IGI Global. doi:10.4018/978-1-5225-1718-4.ch009

Stewart, J. (2017). Introduction Discussion Board Forums in Online Writing Courses Are Essential: No, Really, They Are. In E. Monske & K. Blair (Eds.), *Handbook of Research on Writing and Composing in the Age of MOOCs* (pp. 294–316). Hershey, PA: IGI Global. doi:10.4018/978-1-5225-1718-4.ch018

Stone, J. (2019). Fostering Social Presence on Virtual Learning Teams. In M. Boboc & S. Koç (Eds.), *Student-Centered Virtual Learning Environments in Higher Education* (pp. 134–156). Hershey, PA: IGI Global. doi:10.4018/978-1-5225-5769-2.ch006

Strang, K. D. (2017). Predicting Student Satisfaction and Outcomes in Online Courses Using Learning Activity Indicators. *International Journal of Web-Based Learning and Teaching Technologies*, *12*(1), 32–50. doi:10.4018/IJWLTT.2017010103

Sutha, J. (2018). Exploring the Role of Adult Learning Theory in Understanding Employees' Participation in Non-Mandatory Training. In F. Giuseffi (Ed.), *Emerging Self-Directed Learning Strategies in the Digital Age* (pp. 48–80). Hershey, PA: IGI Global. doi:10.4018/978-1-5225-3465-5.ch004

Tahiri, J. S., Bennani, S., & Idrissi, M. K. (2018). Differentiated Instruction Supporting MOOC: A Pedagogical Framework to Improve the Dropout Rate. In R. Queirós (Ed.), *Emerging Trends, Techniques, and Tools for Massive Open Online Course (MOOC) Management* (pp. 130–154). Hershey, PA: IGI Global. doi:10.4018/978-1-5225-5011-2.ch006

Teine, M. (2018). A Prototypical Participatory Design-Process: Bringing Digital Learning and User Experience Together. In I. Bouchrika, N. Harrati, & P. Vu (Eds.), *Learner Experience and Usability in Online Education* (pp. 36–60). Hershey, PA: IGI Global. doi:10.4018/978-1-5225-4206-3.ch002

Tham, J. C. (2017). Audience, User, Producer: MOOCs as Activity Systems. In E. Monske & K. Blair (Eds.), *Handbook of Research on Writing and Composing in the Age of MOOCs* (pp. 254–277). Hershey, PA: IGI Global. doi:10.4018/978-1-5225-1718-4.ch016

Tlili, A., Essalmi, F., Jemni, M., Kinshuk, & Chen, N.-S. (2018). A Complete Validated Learning Analytics Framework: Designing Issues from Data Preparation Perspective. *International Journal of Information and Communication Technology Education*, *14*(2), 1–16. doi:10.4018/IJICTE.2018040101

Topal, M., & Karaca, O. (2018). Gamification in E-Learning. In R. Queirós (Ed.), *Emerging Trends, Techniques, and Tools for Massive Open Online Course (MOOC) Management* (pp. 79–105). Hershey, PA: IGI Global. doi:10.4018/978-1-5225-5011-2.ch004

Umar, M. A., Shuru, A., Kufena, A. M., Tanko, M. Y., Sambo, A. A., & Hassan, S. A. (2018). Mobile CGPA Monitoring System: A Tool to Guide Self-Directed Learning. In F. Giuseffi (Ed.), *Emerging Self-Directed Learning Strategies in the Digital Age* (pp. 10–21). Hershey, PA: IGI Global. doi:10.4018/978-1-5225-3465-5.ch002

Ünal, E., & Çakır, H. (2019). Use of Dynamic Web Technologies in Collaborative Problem-Solving Method at Community Colleges. In M. Boboc & S. Koç (Eds.), *Student-Centered Virtual Learning Environments in Higher Education* (pp. 185–209). Hershey, PA: IGI Global. doi:10.4018/978-1-5225-5769-2.ch008

Varanasi, M. R., Fischetti, J. C., & Smith, M. W. (2018). Analytics Framework for K-12 School Systems. In E. Mense & M. Crain-Dorough (Eds.), *Data Leadership for K-12 Schools in a Time of Accountability* (pp. 206–233). Hershey, PA: IGI Global. doi:10.4018/978-1-5225-3188-3.ch011

Velliaris, D. M. (2018). An Intervention Program for Advancing the Academic Performance of International Pathway "STAR". In M. Kumar Singh, Z. Zerihun, & N. Singh (Eds.), *Impact of Learning Analytics on Curriculum Design and Student Performance* (pp. 71–95). Hershey, PA: IGI Global. doi:10.4018/978-1-5225-5369-4.ch006

Wani, S. A., Wani, Z. A., & Bhat, A. R. (2019). Identification and Evaluation of Quality of Open Access Journals Cited by Researchers of MIT, CIT and STANFORD. In E. Ossiannilsson (Ed.), *Ubiquitous Inclusive Learning in a Digital Era* (pp. 179–198). Hershey, PA: IGI Global. doi:10.4018/978-1-5225-6292-4.ch008

Wheat, J. (2018). Assessment Literacy Within Middle School-Level Math Professional Learning Communities. In E. Mense & M. Crain-Dorough (Eds.), *Data Leadership for K-12 Schools in a Time of Accountability* (pp. 119–139). Hershey, PA: IGI Global. doi:10.4018/978-1-5225-3188-3.ch007

White, C. C., & Johnson, J. (2018). Change Management in K-12 Education for Data-Driven Decisions: Moving From Professional Judgment to Evidence. In E. Mense & M. Crain-Dorough (Eds.), *Data Leadership for K-12 Schools in a Time of Accountability* (pp. 54–74). Hershey, PA: IGI Global. doi:10.4018/978-1-5225-3188-3.ch004

Willis, J. E. III, & Strunk, V. A. (2017). The Ethics of Machine-Based Learning: Advancing without Losing Humanity. *International Journal of Sociotechnology and Knowledge Development*, *9*(1), 53–66. doi:10.4018/IJSKD.2017010104

Zeirhun, Z. (2018). Learning Analytics: A Critical Review of the Role and Implementation in Educational Institutions. In M. Kumar Singh, Z. Zerihun, & N. Singh (Eds.), *Impact of Learning Analytics on Curriculum Design and Student Performance* (pp. 41–55). Hershey, PA: IGI Global. doi:10.4018/978-1-5225-5369-4.ch004

Zesu, S. (2018). Assessment and Evaluation of Students' Performance Without Learning Analytics. In M. Kumar Singh, Z. Zerihun, & N. Singh (Eds.), *Impact of Learning Analytics on Curriculum Design and Student Performance* (pp. 96–112). Hershey, PA: IGI Global. doi:10.4018/978-1-5225-5369-4.ch007

About the Authors

Paula Miller is a Research Affiliate with the Center for Educational and Instructional Technology with the University of Phoenix. She has been an oncology program manager for Southern California Medical Centers. In addition, she is a Certified Health Education Specialist and has received the Antronette Yancey Physical Activity/Fitness Award from the Southern California Public Health Association. Further, Dr. Miller is a reviewer and evaluator of courses for Blackboard, an educational technology company for online education.

James Connelly is a retired professor from higher education with more than 30 years' experience in the production of instructional media for the health sciences professions. He has been an Online facilitator and a doctoral chairman for more than 16 years with the University of Phoenix. He is also a Research Affiliate with the Center for Educational and Instructional Technology with the University of Phoenix. Before that, he was a radio operator in the Navy, a telecommunications specialist for the CIA, and a Radio Officer in the Merchant Marine (with the National Oceanographic and Atmospheric Administration). While with the University of Tennessee Health Science Center in Memphis, between 1984 and 2000, he produced almost 800 major productions for a variety of clients, many of which were multinational companies.

Index

N

O

P

R

S

T

U

W

www.ingramcontent.com/pod-product-compliance
Ingram Content Group UK Ltd.
Pitfield, Milton Keynes, MK11 3LW, UK
UKHW050945290926
15470UKWH00005B/1643